365 DAYS OF GREEN SMOOTHIE

Emma Katie

Check out more books by Emma Katie at:
www.amazon.com/author/emmakatie

ISBN-13: 978-1539581451

Contents

Introduction

This book is all about smoothies. In this book, you will find out 365 awesome and interesting recipes of smoothies. It can be said that this book is a proper guide of smoothie recipes and no other quality recipes can be found on internet or in other source than this book. We can say this confidently because 365 is a huge number. All the recipes in this book are well-managed, cost effective and easy to perform. It won't cause you a lot of time or money to make smoothies using these recipes. Before we jump into the recipes, here are some key information for you. What is smoothie? The name smoothie came from the idea of smooth property. So, the main thing behind smoothie is, it has to be smooth and easy to digest. This is the reason why smoothies are mostly liquid. Smoothie is a blended form of fruits. Though this is the traditional definition of smoothie, smoothie is not limited to this. Smoothies can contain chocolate, peanut butter and things like that. It can also contain sweetened beverages in it. The basic idea of smoothie began in Brazil in the era of 1940s. A famous book was published at that time named "Banana Smoothie" which is known as the first ever smoothie book. At that time, everything that is made in blender was considered as smoothie. The director of the Juice and Smoothie Association then announced that smoothies are those juices that are made of fruits. Smoothies started to become popular in a quick time and it became available in all restaurants in other pubs from 1960s. So, now you know a lot about smoothies. No, you are not yet ready to jump into the recipes. You need to know about green smoothies now. Till now what we were discussing was about general smoothies but this book is not about that. The title of this book suggests that this book is about green smoothies. So, let's know what green smoothies are. The name "Green Smoothie" says it all. Green smoothies are those smoothies which are made of green fruits and vegetables. You cannot use a food color in a green smoothie. They are better than the regular smoothies in terms of taste, nutrition value and what not. That is why this book is all about green smoothies.

Why Green Smoothies?

Green vegetables and fruits are considered as the most healthy food available on the planet. This is the main reason behind saying green smoothie as the best smoothie. Taking a green smoothie is obviously better than eating salad with a dish. There are reasons behind this. The most important reason is, you get to eat a lot of greens when you take a smoothie. It is not possible to take so much of healthy ingredients with salad. So, Smoothie is obviously the best option. Green smoothies will never cause you fat related problems. They are smart and healthy. You won't get affected by stomach related problems no matter how much you take green smoothies and they are great against heart related diseases. So, do not waste time and make taking green smoothie a habit. There are people who will tell you that green smoothies do not taste as good as the regular smoothies. Yes, this can be true to some extend but there are lots of options for you to choose from. If you don't like one smoothie then do not waste your time there. Simply move to another one and it is guaranteed that you will like at least hundred recipes from the 365 recipes of this book. Green smoothies are full of vitamins and minerals. It will satisfy your hunger and the nutrition level at the same time. Here are a few reasons that why you should choose green smoothies.

1. Green smoothies have great nutrition value. It will not let you starve for nutrition at all.

2. You don't have to face problems related to digestion. Green smoothies can be digested easily and it won't give you any pain or trouble.

3. Green smoothies are not only juice but also food as they contain fiber. So, it will kill your hunger level and it will give you the necessary amount of fiber that you need.

4. Green smoothies are a great way to nourish your body. Taking one cup of green smoothie will give you a great feeling and if you take it regularly then your body will be properly nourished.

5. It doesn't take much time to make green smoothies and it takes almost no time to clean the thrash up.

6. Children love green smoothies and it does not have any age barrier. Everyone can try it.

7. When you take green smoothie, you reduce the consumption of oil and salt in your body which is good.

8. If you find green smoothies tasty and if you make it a habit then you will end up having a great health.

There are other benefits such as green smoothies can be stored for a longer time and other reasons. The main thing is, green smoothies are surely one of the best categories of food items of all time.

365 days of Green Smoothie Recipes

Blast of an Island

Ingredients:

1 banana- small sized (ripe and peeled)
Celery- 1 rib
Cucumber- 1/4th
Pineapple- 1 cup
Parsley- 1 handful
Ginger – ½ inch or less
Coconut water- 1 to 2 cups

Directions:

1. Simply add everything in the blender. As you already used coconut water, you don't need to use water separately.
2. Turn your blender on and blend it till it gets mixed. Take a mug and collect the smoothie from the blender.
3. Use one or two piece of ice if needed.

Enjoy.

Cream of Green

Ingredients:

1 piece of avocado (pits have to be removed)
1 frozen banana (small to medium size)
1 piece of orange
½ to 1 cup of spinach
1 to 2 cup of vanilla milk- unsweetened

Directions:

1. Turn your blender on. This can be done without blender too but that will cause you much time.
2. Remove the pits of the avocado. It has to be peeled.
3. Put everything in the blender and make the juice for at least 2 minutes.

Enjoy.

Cleanse from Tropicana

Ingredients:

Fresh pineapple- 1 cup
Banana- 1 piece
Ginger- 1 inch piece
Spinach- 2 handful
Water- 1 Cup

Directions:

1. Turn your blender on. You can use regular water or coconut water. It is totally up to you.
2. If you use coconut water then that has to be unpasteurized.
3. Pour everything into the blender. Make sure that the banana you are using is ripe and peeled.
4. Juice it for 2 minutes.

Enjoy.

Banana Berry Smoothie

Ingredients:

Spinach- 2 cups
Banana- 1 piece
Mixed berries0 3/4th cup
Raw nuts- ¼th cup
Water- 1-2 cups

Directions:

1. Make sure the banana is ripe. It should be peeled too.
2. You can also use strawberries or blueberries in it. Go for sunflower seeds or flax seeds for the raw seed category.
3. You can also use coconut water if you don't want to use the normal one.
4. Now simply put everything in the blender and switch it on. Blend it for two minutes.

Enjoy.

Strawberry with Lemonade

Ingredients:

Kiwi – 1 piece
Fresh strawberry- 3/4th cup
¼ - ½ cup pineapple
Lemon- ½ cup
Spinach- 2 Cups
Water- 1.5 cup

Directions:

1. You can use coconut water instead of regular water if you want. The lemon has to be peeled.
2. The kiwi should also be peeled. Now put everything on the blender and switch it on.
3. Blend it for two and a half minutes. Take it off.

Enjoy.

The Glowing Smoothie

Ingredients:

Organic lettuce- 1 piece
1.5 cup water
Organic spinach – ½ head
Apple- 1 piece
Pear- 1 piece
Banana- 1 piece
Lemon juice- ½ tbsp.

Directions:

1. Simply put water in blender. The next task is to place spinach in it. The trick here is to start slow and speed up.
2. Start the blender in a low speed and then slowly increase the speed and mix it till it gets smooth.
3. When you are increasing the speed, slowly add everything into it. Add the lemon juice at the end.
4. It should be done within 5 minutes.

Enjoy.

Fight to be Well Smoothie

Ingredients:

Kale- 3 stalks
Lettuce – 3 leaves
Coconut water- 1 cup
Banana- 1 piece
Blueberries
Hemp Seeds- 1 tsp
Chia Seeds- 1 tsp
Bee Pollen- 1 tsp
Maca Powder- 1 tsp
Spirulina- 1 tsp

Directions:

1. The making Directions is not tough for this recipe. Simply put everything in your blender at once.
2. Then switch it on and make the smoothie. That is it.

Enjoy.

Powder of Green Smoothie

Ingredients:

Oat Milk- 1 cup
Coconut Water- 1 cup
Spirulina- 1 tsp
Flaxseed meal- 2 tsp
Coconut oil- 1 tbsp
Berries- 1/4th cup
Probiotics- 1tsp
Organic yoghurt- 2 tbsp
Cinnamon
Stevie- 2 drops

Directions:

1. Turn your blender on. Make sure that the coconut oil that you are using is organic. Also, the yoghurt should also be organic.
2. You should not use much of cinnamon. Only a pinch will be enough.
3. Simply put everything in the blender and turn it on.
4. Blend it for 3 minutes and serve.

Enjoy

Renewal Smoothie

Ingredients:

Spinach- 1 bunch
Mint- 1 handful
Parsley- 1 handful
Lemon juice- 1tbsp.
Lettuce Leaves
Stalks- 4 celery
Cucumber- 1 piece
Ginger- 1 piece
Ice- 5 cubes

Directions:

1. Make sure that the spinach is English and the ginger is peeled properly. Turn the motor on and pour everything on it.
2. Do not put ice cubes in the blender. You have to put ice cubes on the top of the smoothie to get a cool feeling.
3. Try to sip it slowly to get extra taste.

Enjoy.

Greeny Green- Beginner's Luck

Ingredients:

Spinach- 2 cup
Water- 2 Cup
Mango- 1 piece
Pineapple- 1 Cup
Banana- 2 piece

Directions:

1. The process is easy. Make sure the spinach is fresh and tightly packed.
2. Now turn the blender on and juice it for at least 3 minutes.
3. Use ice to make it cool.

Enjoy.

Cilantro with Mango Detox

Ingredients:

Spinach- ½ cup
Cilantro- ½ cup
Mango- ½ cup
Water- 2 cups
Pineapple- 1 cup
Avocado- ½

Directions:

1. It is a simple one to make. The firs thing that you need to do is to blend the spinach and cilantro with water.
2. It has to be smooth so blend it until it gets smoother.
3. Now add the left items and blend again.

Enjoy.

Limeade Green Smoothie

Ingredients:

Spinach- ½ cup
Cilantro- ½ cup
Water- 2 cups
Banana- 3 pieces
Lime- 1 pieces
Ginger- 1 inch

Directions:

1. Make sure that everything that you are using are fresh. Otherwise you won't get the exact taste that you should get.
2. Now blend the spinach and cilantro with water till it gets smooth.
3. Now you can add the remaining items and can blend it again till it becomes smoothie.

Enjoy.

Strawberry with Blueberry and banana

Ingredients:

Spinach- 2 cups
Water- 3/4th cup
Orange juice- 3/4th cup
Strawberry- 1 cup
Blueberry- 1 cup
Banana- 2 piece

Directions:

1. Turn your blender on and blend orange juice with spinach. Remember to put water in the blender before putting in the orange juice.
2. Now add the other juice and blend it again for two minutes. You can make this smoothie cold in two ways.
3. Either you can use frozen food or you can also use ice. It is up to you.

Enjoy.

Green Chocolate Cherry

Ingredients:

Cherry- 2 cup
Banana- 2 piece
Cacao Powder- 3tbs
Almond Milk- 2 Cups
Spinach- 2 cups

Directions:

1. Take the spinach and mix it with almond milk. The spinach needs to be fresh and the milk needs to be unsweetened.
2. Now put everything in the blender and blend for three minutes. You will be done.

Enjoy.

Dream Coconut Smoothie

Ingredients:

Spinach- 2 cups
Coconut water- 1 cup

Grape- 2 cups
Peaches- 2 piece

Directions:

1. You need to turn on your blender first. The next task is to blend spinach and coconut till they get smooth.
2. Then simply put the other ingredients in blender and blend again for 2 minutes. It will be done.

Enjoy.

Luck of Newbies

Ingredients:

Pineapple- 1 cup
Mango- 1 piece
Banana- 2 piece
Water- 2 cups
Spinach- 2 cups

Directions:

1. There is a trick in this recipe. You need to blend the spinach and the water together first and you can add other ingredients only after blending those two separately.
2. Blend everything for 3 minutes.
3. Take it out and enjoy. That's it.

Smoothie of Pomegranate

Ingredients:

Banana- 1 piece
Pomegranate seeds- 1 cup
Water- 1 cup
Orange juice- 1 cup
Spinach- 2 cup

Directions:

1. The first task is to blend the spinach and orange juice with the presence of water. Blend these things for two minutes.
2. Then join the other ingredients in it and blend again.

3. Blend it for two minutes. Take it out and serve.
Enjoy

Butter and Jelly Smoothie

Ingredients:

Red grapes- 2 cups
Banana- 2 pieces
Almond butter- 4tbs
Spinach- 2 cups
Almond milk- 2 cups

Directions:

1. Turn your blender on. Now blend the spinach and almond milk in it. Do not mix other things initially.
2. Now add the other items in it.
3. Use frozen grapes to make the whole thing cool.
4. Make sure that you are using unsweetened almond milk and fresh spinach.

Smoothie of Kiwi Berry

Ingredients:

Blueberry- 1 cup
Mixed berry- 1 cup
Banana- 1 piece
Kiwi- 1 piece
Avocado- ½ amount
Spinach- 2 cups

Directions:

1. Firstly blend the spinach and water till it get smoothed.
2. The next task is to add the other ingredients in the blender.
3. Now blend it again for 2-3 minutes. It will be done.
Enjoy

Grape Green Smoothie

Ingredients:

Cantaloupe- ½ of amount
Grapes- 1 cup
Coconut oil- 2 tbs
Water- ½ cup
Almond milk- 1 cup
Spinach- 2 cup

Directions:

1. Pour water in the blender and place spinach and almond milk in it.
2. Make sure the almond milk is unsweetened.
3. Now add the other items in the blender and blend again for 3 minutes.
4. Use a frozen ingredient to make it cool.

Enjoy

Peachy Strawberry Green Smoothie

Ingredients:

Strawberry- 1 cup
Peach- 2 cup
Almond milk- 2 cups
Bok choy- 2 cups

Directions:

1. Make sure the almond milk is unsweetened. Turn the blender on and put bok choy and almond milk in it.
2. Now blend it for two minutes.
3. Now you can put other ingredients in blender. Blend everything for 2 minutes.

Enjoy

Mango with Ginger Smoothie

Ingredients:

Lemon- 1 piece
Mango- 3 cup
Ginger- 1 inch

Cucumber- 1 piece
Water- 2 cups
Parsley- 1 cup
Celery- 1 cup

Directions:

1. You have to blend two things separately.

2. The first task is to blend parsley, celery and water till they get smooth.

3. Then you have to add the other items. Now blend it again. That is it.

Enjoy

Colada Pina Green Smoothie

Ingredients:

Almond Milk- ½ cup
Coconut water- ½ cup
Pineapple- 3 cups
Coconut flakes- 2tbs
Spinach- 2 cups

Directions:

1. Make sure that the almond milk is unsweetened and the pineapple is fresh. Now blend the almond milk, spinach and coconut water in blender.

2. Do not mix other stuffs initially.

3. Now after you are done with blending these things, add the other ingredients. Save some flakes to use that later.

Enjoy.

Cherry with Berry Green

Ingredients:

Mixed berry- 1 cup
Cherry- 1 cup
Banana- 1 cup
Water- 2 cup
Spinach- 2 cup

Directions:

1. Firstly, take the spinach and water and blend them together.
2. Now add the other things into the blender and blend it again. Use a frozen fruit to make the smoothie cool.
3. Remember that you need to take out cherry pits before you make the smoothie.

Enjoy.

Smoothie of Beginner's

Ingredients:

Mango- 1 cup
Banana- 1 piece
Pineapple- 1 cup
Water- 2 cups
Carrots- 2 piece
Spinach- ½ cup

Directions:

1. Take spinach, carrot and water and blend them for two minutes.
2. Now you can add the other ingredients in the blender.
3. Blend again for two minutes. Remember to use a frozen fruit so that the smoothie becomes a cold one.

Enjoy.

Smoothie of Spa Skin

Ingredients:

Coconut water- 2 cup
Pineapple- 2 cup
Spinach- 2 cup
Avocado- 1 piece

Directions:

1. It is very easy to make this smoothie. Simply turn your blender on and blend spinach in coconut water.
2. Then add the other items and blend the whole thing again. You can use a frozen fruit so that the smoothie gets cold.

Enjoy.

Twist of Strawberry

Ingredients:

Kiwi- 2 piece
Banana- 1 piece
Lemon- 1 piece
Strawberry- 2 cup
Orange juice- 2 cup
Kale with dandelion green- 2 cup

Directions:

1. The first task is to turn on the blender and blend kale with dandelion green and orange juice.
2. Now you can add the other items in the blender. Now blend the whole thing again for two minutes.
3. Make sure that the dandelion and kale are fresh enough. You can also use the kiwi skin later on the top.

Enjoy.

Berry full of Protein

Ingredients:

Almond Milk- 2 cups
Strawberry- 1 cup
Banana- 1 piece
Almond- ½ cup
Spinach- 2 cup

Directions:

1. First take spinach in water and blend it perfectly. Then add the other ingredients and blend again for two minutes.
2. You can use ice later to make it cold.
3. You can also use a frozen fruit to make it cold. It is up to you.

Enjoy.

Sunshine Smoothie

Ingredients:

Naval Orange- 3-4 piece
Pineapple- 3 to 4 cup
Collard- 1 cup
Spinach- 1 cup

Directions:

1. The main task here is to squeeze the orange to make the juice. Then put the juice in blender and blend it with spinach and collard.
2. Remember that you haven't put pineapple yet. Now it is the time.
3. Take pineapple and chop it properly before you put it in blender.
4. Blend everything for two minutes. Take it out and put ice before serving.
Enjoy.

Banana and Kale Smoothie

Ingredients:

Kale- 2 cups
Banana- 3 piece
Avocado- 1/4th
Water- 2 cups

Directions:

1. Simply turn your blender on and blend kale in water.
2. Make sure that the kale is properly smoothed.
3. Now put other ingredients in blender and blend again.
Enjoy.

Doctor Cranberry Smoothie

Ingredients:

Cranberry- 1 cup
Orange- 2 piece
Banana- 2 piece
Water- 1 cup
Kale- 2 cup

Directions:

1. Take kale and blend it in water till it gets smooth.
2. Then add the other ingredients in blender and blend again.
3. Make sure that the orange is properly peeled and the kale that you are using is fresh.

Enjoy.

Fight with Radical Smoothie

Ingredients:

Spinach- 2 cups
Blueberry- ½ cup
Apple- 1 piece
Lime- ½ part
Cantaloupe- 2 cups
Water- optional
Mint- 1 sprig

Directions:

1. Make sure that the cantaloupe is ripe and rind properly.
2. Now put spinach with mint and cantaloupe in blender.
3. Turn it on and blend it till it gets smoothed. Then add the other ingredients and blend it again.

Enjoy.

Popsicle of Strawberry and Mint

Ingredients:

spinach- 1.5 cup
Mint- ½ cup
Strawberry- 16oz
Date Syrup/honey- 1/4th cup
Coconut milk- ¼ cup

Directions:

1. Make sure that the strawberry is frozen and cold. It will make the smoothie cold.
2. Firstly, blend mint with spinach and coconut milk. Make sure that it is properly

smoothed.

3. Now add the remaining items and blend it again. You can run cold water over popsicle molds to slide pops out.

Enjoy.

Green, Sweet and Pear Smoothie

Ingredients:

Almond milk- 2 cup
Pears- 4 piece
banana- 1 piece
Cinnamon- 1 tsp
Spinach- 2 cup

Directions:

1. Take spinach and almond milk and blend them nicely. Then add the remaining items and blend it again for two minutes.

2. This smoothie can be served to two people so if you want it only for your own then use half of every ingredients.

Enjoy.

Green Life Smoothie

Ingredients:

Almond milk- 2 cup
Spinach- 2 cup
Sweet Potato- 1 cup
Mango- 2 cup
Cinnamon- 1tsp
Nutmeg- 1 tsp
Water- 1/4th cup

Directions:

1. Take spinach and blend it with almond milk. Make sure the milk is unsweetened.

2. Now add the other ingredients in blender and blend it for two minutes.

3. You can always use ice or a frozen fruit to make it cold.

Enjoy.

Pineapple Crash Smoothie

Ingredients:

Kale- 2 cup
Water- 2 cup
Pineapple- 2 cup
Coconut oil- 2 tbsp
Banana- 1 piece

Directions:

1. Firstly, turn on the blender and blend kale and coconut oil in water till they get smoothed.
2. Then add the other items and blend it again.

Enjoy.

Kale Cooler Smoothie

Ingredients:

Kale- ½ cup
Water- ½ cup
Banana- 2 piece
Lime- 1 piece
Cranberry juice- ½ cup
Blood Orange- 2 piece

Directions:

1. Firstly, take a kale and cranberry juice and blend them with water. Make sure that the oranges are peeled.
2. Now put everything in the same blender and blend again.

Enjoy.

Greeny Cherry Smoothie

Ingredients:

Kale- 2 cup
Almond milk- 2 cup
Cherry- 1 cup
Mango mix- 2 cup

Directions:

1. The Directions of making Greeny cherry is extremely simple.
2. Just turn your blender on and put everything in it at once. As always, you have to make sure that the almond milk is unsweetened.
3. Blend everything for two minutes and enjoy.

That's it.

Coco-Cherry Smoothie

Ingredients:

Kale-2 cup
Coconut milk- 2 cup
Cherry- 2 cup
Blueberry- 1 cup

Directions:

1. Before you turn the blender on, make sure that the coconut milk is unsweetened.
2. Now turn your blender on and put everything in it. Blend it as long as you want.
3. Make sure that everything got properly smoothed.

Enjoy.

Clean your Skin Smoothie

Ingredients:

Spinach- 2 cup
Pineapple- 2 cup
Water- 2 cup
Avocado- 1 piece
Kale- 2 cup

Directions:

1. The kale and the spinach will make this smoothie green. First of all, make sure that the coconut water is unsweetened.
2. Then add everything in blender and blend for two minutes.
3. Then simply take it out, use ice and serve.

Enjoy.

Cherry with Kale Smoothie

Ingredients:

Kale- 2 cup
Almond milk- 2 cup
Pineapple- 2 cup
Mango mix- 2 cup
Cherry- 1 cup

Directions:

1. You don't need both pineapple and mango for this smoothie. You can use any one of them.
2. You have to use unsweetened almond milk.
3. Put everything in blender and turn it on.
4. Blend everything for two- three minutes.
5. Take it out and use ice to make it cold.

Enjoy.

Baby Chard Green Smoothie

Ingredients:

Baby chard- 2 cups
Water- 2 cups
Blueberry- 1 cup
Raspberry- 1 cup
Pineapple- 1 cup
Mango mix- 1 cup

Directions:

1. You don't need both pineapple and mango mix. You can use any of them.
2. Simply turn your blender on and put everything in it at once.
3. Juice it for two minutes.
4. Take it out and use ice to make it cool.

Enjoy.

Vitamin Mixture

Ingredients:

Spinach- 2 cups
Almond milk- 2 cups
Orange- 1 piece
Banana- 1 piece
Pineapple- 2 cups

Directions:

1. The pineapples have to be frozen. This is how the smoothie will be a cold one. You cannot drink a hot smoothie.
2. The almond milk needs to be unsweetened.
3. Take almond milk, spinach, banana and orange and put them in your blender.
4. Turn your blender on and blend them for three minutes.
5. Now put pineapples in it and blend again for two minutes. This will make the smoothie cold.
6. Take it out. It will serve two people.

Enjoy.

Breeze of Freshness

Ingredients:

Spinach- 2 cups
Water- 1.5 cup
Orange- 2 piece
Mango- ½ cup
Pineapple- ½ cup
Banana- 1 piece

Directions:

1. Make sure the spinach is fresh. Otherwise the whole smoothie will taste bad.
2. Oranges have to be peeled before you put them in blender.
3. Take orange, pineapple and banana and put them in blender. Blend them for two to three minutes. Make sure that they mixed properly.
4. Now add spinach in it and extra water if needed. Blend again for two to three minutes.
5. You can either use frozen pineapple and orange or you can also use ice to make it cold.

Enjoy.

Leafy Green Smoothie

Ingredients:

Spinach- 2 cups
Water/Coconut water- 2 cups
Banana- 1 piece
Mango- 1 cup
Peach- 1 piece

Directions:

1. Make sure that the banana and mango are frozen. It will make the smoothie cold.
2. Put everything in blender at once. You don't need to use both coconut water and regular water. Use any of them.
3. Blend it for four minutes.
4. Take it out.

Enjoy.

Breeze of Citrus

Ingredients:

Spinach- 2 cups
Orange- 2 piece
Mango- ½ cup
Pineapple- ½ cup
Banana- 1 piece

Directions:

1. The Directions is extremely simple. Put everything in your blender at once and turn it on.
2. You don't have to worry about any other thing.
3. Use ice later if you want to make it cold.

Enjoy.

Berry Protein with Bash

Ingredients:

Spinach- 2 cups
Coconut juice- 2 cups
Strawberries- 1 cup
Blueberry- 1 cup
Banana- 1 piece
Almond- ½ cup

Directions:

1. Make sure that the almond is soaked properly. Take 1 cup coconut juice instead of two if you want to make it for one person.
2. Turn your blender on and put everything in it at once.
3. Make sure that the blueberries and strawberries are frozen before they are put in blender.
4. It will make the smoothie cold.

Enjoy.

Beery Melon

Ingredients:

Spinach- 2 cups
Water- 1 cup
Watermelon- 2 cups
Berry- 1 cup

Directions:

1. Turn your blender on and put the frozen berries in it. The frozen berries will make the smoothie cold.
2. Blend everything for 3 minutes.

Enjoy

Peachy Cobbler of Blackberry

Ingredients:

Spinach- 2 cups
Almond milk- 2 cups

Blackberry- 2 cups
Peach- 1 piece
Flax seed- 2 tbsp.
Cinnamon- ½ tbsp

Directions:

1. Put everything in blender and turn it on.

2. Blend it for two minutes.

Enjoy

Almond Mania

Ingredients:

Almond- 1 piece
Lemon juice- ½ tea spoon
Water- 3 cups
Vanilla- 1 teaspoon
Nut Milk Bag- 1 nut

Directions:

1. Put everything in blender and turn it on.

2. Blend it for 3 minutes.

Enjoy

Fresca of Watermelon

Ingredients:

Spinach- 2 cups
Water- 1 cup
Watermelon- ½ cup
Strawberry- ½ cup
Ginger- 1 inch

Directions:

1. Wash everything before you start.

2. Blend everything for three minutes.

Enjoy

Cherry of Almond

Ingredients:

Spinach- 2 cups
Almond Milk- 2 cups
Cherries- 2 cups
Banana- 1 piece
Cinnamon- ½ tbsp

Directions:

1. Make sure that the milk is unsweetened.
2. Put everything in blender and turn it on.
3. Blend it for three minutes.

Enjoy

Cake of Pineapple

Ingredients:

Spinach- 2 cups
Almond milk- 2 cups
Pineapple- 1 cup
Cherry- 1 cup
Banana- 1 piece

Directions:

1. Make sure the cherries are pitted.
2. Make sure the almond milk is unsweetened.
3. Turn your blender on and blend it for three minutes.

Enjoy

Leafy Green Juice

Ingredients:

Leafy Greens- 2 cups
Liquid green- 2 cup
Any fruit- 3 cups

Directions:

1. Simply turn your blender on and put everything in it.
2. Blend it for three minutes.

Enjoy.

Greeny Coconut Smoothie

Ingredients:

Coconut milk- 1 cup
Water- 1 cup
Blueberry- 1 cup
Flax seed- 1 cup
Goji berry- 1 tbsp.
Spinach- 1 handful
Banana- 2 pieces

Directions:

1. Wash spinach and other items properly and turn the blender on.
2. Blend it for three minutes.

Enjoy

Smoothie of Coco

Ingredients:

Kale- 2 cups
Coconut milk- 2 cups
Cherries- 2 cup
Blueberries- 1 cup

Directions:

1. Put everything in blender and turn it on.
2. Blend for 4 minutes.

Enjoy

Smoothie of Almond

Ingredients:

Kale- 2 cups
Almond milk- 2 cups
Cherry- 2 cup
Blueberry- 1 cup

Directions:

1. Simply put everything in your blender and turn it on.
2. Blend the items for 4 minutes.
Enjoy

Dream of Coconut Smoothie

Ingredients:

Peach- 1 piece
Grape- 2 cups
Spinach- 2 cups
Coconut water- 1 cup

Directions:

1. Simply put everything in blender and turn it on.
2. Blend it for three minutes.
Enjoy

Popsicle of Pumpkin

Ingredients:

Pumpkin- 1 piece
Almond milk- 2 cup
Leafy greens- 2 cups
Banana- 2 piece
Frozen mango- 1 cup
Pumpkin spice- 1 tsp

Directions:

1. Simply put everything in your blender and mix them with a spoon.

2. Now turn your blender on and blend for 4 minutes.
Enjoy

Smoothie of Berry

Ingredients:

Banana- 1 piece
Strawberry- 2 piece
Blueberry- 2 pieces
Spinach- 2 cups
Water/Coconut water- 1.5 cup

Directions:

1. Take one frozen fruit to make the smoothie cold.
2. Pour everything in blender and turn it on.
3. Blend it for 4 minutes.
Enjoy

Bowl of Smoothie

Ingredients:

Avocado- ½ piece
Baby Spinach- 1 cup
Kiwi- 1 piece
Frozen Banana- 1 piece
Almond milk- 1 cup
Chia seeds- 1tbsp.
Virgin coconut oil- 1tbsp.

Directions:

1. Simply put everything in blender and blend for 5 minutes.
2. Take it out and pour it in a bowl.
Enjoy

Green of Morning

Ingredients:

Cucumber- 1 piece

Celery- 1 piece
Apple- 1 piece
Ginger- 1 piece
Spinach- 1 handful
Mango- 1 cup

Directions:

1. Take everything in your blender. Make sure that they are cut uniformly.
2. Turn the blender on and blend for 4 minutes.

Enjoy

Crush of Carrot

Ingredients:

Kale- 2.5 cup
Water- 1.5 cup
Banana- ½ piece
Baby Carrot- 2-3 pieces
Chia seed- 1tbsp

Directions:

1. Turn your blender on and put everything in it.
2. Blend for 3.5 minutes.

Enjoy

Jubilee of Coconut Smoothie

Ingredients:

Mixed fruits- 1.5 cups
Cherry- ½ cup
Coconut oil- 2 tbsp.
Coconut flakes- 2tbsp.
Spinach- 2 cup
Coconut water- 2 cup

Directions:

1. Put everything at once in your blender. Turn it on.
2. Blend it for 5 minutes.

Enjoy

Spice of Pumpkin

Ingredients:

Raw pumpkin- 1 cup
Almond milk0 ½ cup
Pumpkin pie- 2 tsp.
Carrot- 1 piece
Spinach- 2 cups
Banana- 2 pieces

Directions:

1. Place all the ingredients in you blender and turn it on.
2. Serve with some ice cubes.

Green Potato Smoothie

Ingredients:

Sweet Potato- 1 cup
Frozen mango- 2 cups
Baby spinach- 3 cup
Almond milk- 2 cups
Water-1/4th cup
Cinnamon- 1tsp
Nutmeg- 1tsp

Directions:

1. Cut the vegetables and fruits into cubes to fit in the bender.
2. Blend it for around 3 minutes

Power Booster Smoothie

Ingredients:

Kale- 2/3 cups
Light coconut milk- 1 cup
Water- 1 cup
Frozen mango- 1 cup
Persimmons- 2 piece

Banana- 1 piece
Shredded coconut- 3tbsp

Directions:

1. Place all the ingredients in you blender and turn it on.
2. Blend it for around 3 minutes.

Cranberry Cleanser

Ingredients:

Kale- 2 cups
Water- 1 cup
Ice cubes- 6 pieces
Cranberry- 1 cup
Orange- 2 (peeled)
Banana- 2 piece
Flax seed- 4tbsp.

Directions:

1. Turn your blender on and put everything in it.
Enjoy.

Hydrating Grape Smoothie

Ingredients:

Spinach- 2 cup
Avocado- 1 cup
Banana- 1 cup
Mango- 1 cup
frozen grape- 1 cup
coconut water- 2 cups
Flax seed- 4tbsp.

Directions:

1. Cut the vegetables and fruits into cubes to fit in the bender.
2. Use unsweetened coconut water.

Sweet Pear

Ingredients:

Pear- 4 pieces
Banana- 1 piece
Baby spinach- 2 cups
Vanilla almond milk- 2 cups
Cinnamon- 1tsp

Directions:

1. Put everything at once in your blender.
2. Turn it on and blend for two minutes.
Enjoy

Fun with Vanilla

Ingredients:

Vanilla beans- 2 piece
Vegetable glycerine- 4oz

Directions:

1. Blend it for around 2 minutes.
2. Serve with some ice cubes.

Tasty Smoothie

Ingredients:

Banana- 1 piece
Frozen Mango- 2 cup
Spinach- 3 cups
Cold Water- 4 cups

Directions:

1. Chop the vegetables.
2. Blend it for around 2.5 minutes.

Magic Smoothie

Ingredients:

Kale- 2 cups
Coconut water- 2 cups
Cucumber- ½ piece
Pear- 1 ripe
Mango- 1 ripe
Peaches- 1 cup

Directions:

1. Cut the vegetables and fruits into cubes to fit in the bender
2. Place all the ingredients in you blender and turn it on.

Berry of Melon

Ingredients:

Spinach- 2 cups
Water- 1 cup
Watermelon- 2 cups
Mixed berry- 1 cup

Directions:

1. Cut the vegetables and fruits into cubes to fit in the bender.
2. Serve and enjoy.

Green can be mean smoothie

Ingredients:

Apple- 2 piece
Cucumber- 1 piece
Celery- 4 stalk
Ginger root- 1 thumb
Kale- around six leafs
Lemon- ½ piece

Directions:

1. Place all the ingredients in your blender and turn it on.

2. Blend it for around 3 minutes.

Any time Smoothie

Ingredients:

Apple- 2 piece
Cucumber- 1 piece
Orange- 1 cup
Kale- four leafs
Celery- 4 stalks

Directions:

1. Cut the vegetables and fruits into cubes to fit in the bender.
2. Serve with some ice cubes.

Lemonade Smoothie

Ingredients:

Cucumber- 1 piece
Kale- four leafs
Spinach- 2 leafs
Lemon- 1 piece

Directions:

1. Place all the ingredients in your blender and turn it on.
2. Blend it for around 3 minutes.
3. Serve with some ice cubes.

Weegman's Smoothie

Ingredients:

Root of Beet- 2 pieces
Celery
Spinach- 1 handful
Spirulina- dried

Directions:

1. Chop the vegetables.

2. Place all the ingredients in your blender
3. Blend it for around 3 minutes.

Tangy Smoothie

Ingredients:

Carrot- 2 piece
Beet root- 1 cup
Celery- 1 cup
Spinach- 1 handful
Lime- 1 cup
Ginger root- 1 cup
pepper- half tsp.

Directions:

1. Place all the ingredients in your blender and turn it on.
2. Blend it for around 3 minutes.
3. Serve and enjoy.

Workout Smoothie

Ingredients:

Dandelion Greens- 1 cup
Lemon- half piece
Celery- 1 cup
Kale- 1 cup
Apple- 1 piece

Directions:

1. Remove the seeds from the lemon and peel it properly.
2. Place all the ingredients in your blender
3. Blend it for around 2 minutes.
4. Serve with a lemon slice.

Kale-cium Smoothie

Ingredients:

Apple- 1 piece

Carrot- 1 piece
Kale- 2 handful
Pepper- 1 cup
Cilantro- half cup
Collard greens- half cup

Directions:

1. Cut the vegetables and fruits into cubes to fit in the bender
2. Blend it for around 3 minutes.
3. Serve with some ice cubes.

Morning Smoothie

Ingredients:

Cabbage- 1 cup
Broccoli- 1 cup
Kale- 1 handful

Directions:

1. Remove the pits from the broccoli.
2. Chop the vegetables nicely.
3. Blend it for around 3 minutes.

Tropical Smoothie

Ingredients:

Mango- 1 big piece
Pineapple- 1 cup
Kale- 2 handful
Orange- half cup

Directions:

1. Remove the seeds from the orange and peel it properly.
2. Place all the ingredients in your blender and turn it on.
3. Serve with a orange slice.

Green Aid Smoothie

Ingredients:

Apple- 1 piece
Celery- 1 handful
Spinach- 1 handful
Kale- 1 cup
Lemon- ½ piece

Directions:

1. Cut the vegetables and fruits into cubes to fit in the bender
2. Remove the seeds from the lemon and peel it properly.
3. Blend it for around 3 minutes.
Enjoy.

Salsa Smoothie

Ingredients:

Tomato- 1 cup
Pepper- 1 cup
Onion- half cup
Garlic- half cup
Salt- 1tsp.

Directions:

1. Place all the ingredients in your blender and turn it on.
2. Blend it for around 3 minutes.
3. Serve with some ice cubes.

Breakfast Smoothie

Ingredients:

carrot- 1 piece
Tomato- 1 cup
Spinach- 1 handful
Pepper- half tsp
Cucumber- half cup

Directions:

1. Turn on your blender and blend all the ingredients until it gets smoothed
2. Serve with some ice cubes.

Asparagus Smoothie

Ingredients:

Celery- 1 cup
Asparagus- 1 cup
Cilantro- 1 cup

Directions:

1. Place all the ingredients in your blender and turn it on.
2. Blend it for around 3 minutes.
3. Serve with some ice cubes.

Lime of Lemon

Ingredients:

Lemon- 1 piece
Asian pears- 2 piece
Green apple- 2 piece
Carrots- 2 piece
Ginger- 1 piece
Cabbage- 2 cups

Directions:

1. Remove the seeds from the lemon and peel it properly.
2. Cut the vegetables and fruits into cubes to fit in the bender.
3. Turn on your blender and blend all the ingredients
4. Serve and enjoy.

Green Salsa with Mango

Ingredients:

Mango- 1 piece
Cucumber- ½ piece

Yellow pepper- ¼ piece
Jalapeno pepper- ½ piece
Green onion- 2 piece
Cilantro- ¼ cup
Lime- ½ piece

Directions:

1. Make sure you are using ripe mango.
2. Turn on your blender and blend all the ingredients until it gets smoothed
3. Serve and enjoy.

Peachy Smoothie

Ingredients:

Spinach- 2 piece
Kale- 8 leafs
Peach- 4 piece
Apple- 1 piece
Lemon- ½ piece

Directions:

1. Cut the vegetables and fruits into cubes to fit in the bender.
2. Blend it for around 3 minutes.
3. Pour into a mug and use some ice cube to make it cool.

Mint mixed fruit Smoothie

Ingredients:

Orange- 2 piece
Grapefruit- ½ piece
Carrot- 1 piece
Celery- 2 stalks
Mint- 1/3 bunch
Spinach- 2 handful

Directions:

1. Remove the seeds from the orange and peel it properly.
2. Turn on your blender and blend all the ingredients until it gets smoothed

3. Serve with some ice cubes.

Berry with Mint

Ingredients:

Blueberry- 2 cups
Kiwi- 2 piece
Strawberry- 16 piece
Mint leafs- 2 cup
spinach- 1 handful

Directions:

1. Place all the ingredients in your blender and turn it on.
2. Pour into a mug and use some ice cube to make it cool.

Lemon with apple

Ingredients:

Apples with skin- 2 piece
Lemon- 1 piece
Ginger- 1"
Spinach- 1 handful

Directions:

1. Turn on your blender and blend all the ingredients until it gets smoothed
2. Serve with some ice cubes.

Alkaline smoothie

Ingredients:

Spinach- 1 cup
Cucumber with skin- ½ piece
Celery- 2 stalks
Carrots- 3 piece
Apple- ½ piece

Directions:

1. Cut the vegetables and fruits into cubes to fit in the bender.

2. Blend it for around 3 minutes.
3. Pour into a mug and use some ice cube to make it cool.
4. Keep the smoothie in an air tight jar in your freeze if you want to store it.

Berry with Merry

Ingredients:

Strawberry- 2 cups
Blueberry- 2 cups
Raspberry- ½ cup
Kale- 2 handful

Directions:

1. You need to remove the stems from the kale
2. Turn on your blender and blend all the ingredients until it gets smoothed.
3. Serve with some ice cubes.

Dew of Melon

Ingredients:

Watermelon- ½ piece
Honeydew- ½ cup
Cantaloupe- ½ cup
Spinach- 1 handful

Directions:

1. Make sure you are using ripe cantaloupe.
2. Place all the ingredients in your blender and turn it on.
3. Blend it for around 3 minutes.
4. You can store the smoothie in your refrigerator for 2 days.

Aloha Smoothie

Ingredients:

Mango- 1 piece
Orange- 1 piece
Pineapple- 1 slice
Papaya- 1 piece

Guava- 3 piece

Directions:

1. Remove the seeds from the orange and peel it properly.
2. Place all the ingredients in your blender and turn it on.
3. Pour into a mug and use some ice cube to make it cool.
4. For getting the highest potency of this smoothie drink this within 15 minutes.

Greeny Green Smoothie

Ingredients:

Spinach- 1 cup
Kale- 2 cups
Parsley- 2 cups
Cucumber- 1 piece
Celery- 3 stalks

Directions:

1. You need to remove the stems from the kale
2. Cut the vegetables into cubes to fit in the bender.
3. Blend it for around 3 minutes.
4. Serve with some ice cubes.

Capple Smoothie

Ingredients:

Cucumber- ½ piece with skin on
Apples- 2 piece with skin on

Directions:

1. Turn on your blender and blend all the ingredients until it gets smoothed.
2. Pour into a mug and use some ice cube to make it cool.

Fun Smoothie

Ingredients:

Carrot- 3 piece

Kale- 1 cup
Broccoli- 2 cup

Directions:

1. Remove the pits from the broccoli.
2. Place all the ingredients in your blender and turn it on.
3. Blend it for around 3 minutes.
4. Keep the smoothie in an air tight jar in your freeze if you want to store it.

Killing Smoothie

Ingredients:

Beet with greens- 1 or 2 piece
Apples- 3 piece with skin on

Directions:

1. Turn on your blender and blend all the ingredients until it gets smoothed.
2. Pour into a mug and use some ice cube to make it cool.

Energy boosting Smoothie

Ingredients:

Apples- 2 piece
Cucumber- ½ piece
Lemon- ½ piece
Kale- ½ cup
Spinach- 1 cup
Celery- ¼ handful
fennel- ¼ bulb
ginger- 1" slice
Romaine lettuce- ¼ head

Directions:

1. You need to remove the stems from the kale and chop the vegetables.
2. Place all the ingredients in your blender and turn it on.
3. Blend it for around 3 minutes.
4. Serve with some ice cubes.

Sweet Green Smoothie

Ingredients:

Cucumber- 1 piece
Carrot- 1 piece
Apple- 1 piece
Parsley- 1/4th
Mint- ½ cup
Celery- 1 stalk
Ginger- ½ inch
Lemon- ½ piece
Spinach- 1 handful

Directions:

1. Cut the vegetables and fruits into cubes to fit in the bender.
2. Blend it for around 3 minutes.

Carrot Mania

Ingredients:

Carrots- 5 piece
Broccoli- 1 piece
Spinach- 1 handful

Directions:

1. Remove the pits from the broccoli.
2. Turn on your blender and blend all the ingredients until it gets smoothed.
3. Pour into a mug and use some ice cube to make it cool.

Papple Smoothie

Ingredients:

Apples- 2 piece
Pears- 2 piece with skin on
Spinach- 2 handful

Directions:

1. Place all the ingredients in your blender and turn it on.

2. Serve with some ice cubes.

Carrot Apple with Lemon Smoothie

Ingredients:

Carrots- 4 piece
Apple- 1 piece
Lemon- 1 piece
Spinach- 1 handful

Directions:

1. Remove the seeds from the lemon and peel it properly.
2. Turn on your blender and blend all the ingredients until it gets smoothed.
3. Keep the smoothie in an air tight jar in your freeze if you want to store it.

Cleanser Smoothie

Ingredients:

Papaya- 1 firm
Ginger root- ¼ inch
Pear- 1 piece
Water- 2 cups

Directions:

1. Make sure you are using ripe fruits.
2. Place all the ingredients in your blender and turn it on.
3. Blend it for around 2 minutes.
4. Pour into a mug and use some ice cube to make it cool.

Kidney cleaning Smoothie

Ingredients:

Celery- 3 stalks
Tomatoes- 2 piece
Lemon- 1 piece
Carrot- 2 piece
Water- 2 cup
Spinach- 2 handful

Directions:

1. Turn on your blender and blend all the ingredients until it gets smoothed.
2. For getting the highest potency of this smoothie drink this within 15 minutes.
3. You can store the smoothie in your refrigerator for 2 days.

Glow for you

Ingredients:

Cucumber- 1 piece
Parsley- ½ bunch
Alfalfa sprouts- 4 oz
fresh mint- 4 sprigs
Water- 2 cup
Spirulina- 2 handful

Directions:

1. Cut the vegetables and fruits into cubes to fit in the bender.
2. Blend it for around 3 minutes
3. Serve with some mint leaves.

Pumper for you

Ingredients:

Grape- 2 bunch
Orange- 6 piece
Lemon- 8 piece
Honey- 1/4th cup
Water- 3 mug
Spinach- 4 handful

Directions:

1. Remove the seeds from the lemon and orange.
2. Use cold water to make the juice cold.
3. Serve and enjoy.

Clean your Stomach Smoothie

Ingredients:

Grape- 1 bunch
Strawberry- 1 basket
Apples- 3piece
Mint- 4 sprigs
Water- 2 cups
Spinach- 3 handful

Directions:

1. Turn on your blender and blend all the ingredients until it gets smoothed.
2. Pour into a mug and use some ice cube to make it cool.
3. Keep the smoothie in an air tight jar in your freeze if you want to store it.

Sweet green Smoothie

Ingredients:

Raspberry- 2 cup
Strawberry- 2 cup
Orange- 1 piece
Apple- 2 piece
Spinach- 3 handful

Directions:

1. Turn on your blender and blend all the ingredients until it gets smoothed.
2. Serve with some ice cubes.

Copy Cat Smoothie

Ingredients:

Tomato- 3 piece
Celery- 3 stalks
Carrot- 5 piece
Beet- 1 piece
Cabbage- 1/4th head
Bell pepper(green)- ½ piece
Spinach- 2 cups
Sweet onion- 1/4th cup

Garlic- ½ clove

Directions:

1. Cut the vegetables and fruits into smaller pieces to fit in the bender
2. Blend it for around 3 minutes.
3. Pour into a mug and use some ice cube to make it cool.

Green mango smoothie

Ingredients:

Green mango- 1 piece
Orange- 1 piece
Papaya- ½ piece
Pineapple- 1/4th piece
Banana- 1 piece

Directions:

1. Use ripe fruits to make this smoothie.
2. Turn on your blender and blend all the ingredients until it gets smoothed.
3. Serve with some ice cubes.

Grapeful Smoothie

Ingredients:

Red grape- 1 cup
Lemon- ½ cup
Orange- 2 cup
Water- 4ounce
Spinach- 4 handful

Directions:

1. Remove the seeds from the lemon and peel it properly.
2. Place all the ingredients in your blender and turn it on
3. Blend it for around 3 minutes.
4. Keep the smoothie in an air tight jar in your freeze if you want to store it.

Apple with Spinach

Ingredients:

Apple- 3 piece
Spinach- 3 cups
Broccoli stems- ½ cup

Directions:

1. Remove the pits from the broccoli.
2. Turn on your blender and blend all the ingredients until it gets smoothed.
3. Serve with some ice cubes.
4. For getting the highest potency of this smoothie drink this within 15 minutes.

Morning Smoothie

Ingredients:

Orange- 2 piece
Grapefruit- 1 piece
Strawberry- 6 frozen piece
Banana- ½ piece
Spinach- 2 cups

Directions:

1. Use ripe fruits to make this smoothie.
2. Place all the ingredients in your blender and turn it on.
3. Blend it for around 2.5 minutes.
4. Serve with some ice cubes.

Love of Melon

Ingredients:

Watermelon- 2 cup
Cantaloupe- 2 cup
Ginger- 1 inch
Spinach- 2 cu

Directions:

1. Cut the vegetables and fruits into smaller pieces to fit in the bender.
2. Blend it for around 3 minutes.
3. Pour into a mug and use some ice cube to make it cool.

Greeny Strawberry with Orange

Ingredients:

Strawberry- ½ cup
Orange juice- 1 cup
Lemon juice- 2tsp
Spinach- 2 cup

Directions:

1. Turn on your blender and blend all the ingredients until it gets smoothed.
2. Serve with some ice cubes.

Tummy Cleaner at home

Ingredients:

Carrots- 4 large piece
Celery- 1 stalk
Apple- 1 piece
Spinach- handful
Lemon juice- ½ cup

Directions:

1. Place all the ingredients in your blender and turn it on.
2. Blend it for around 3 minutes.
3. For getting the highest potency of this smoothie drink this within 15 minutes.
4. You can store the smoothie in your refrigerator for 2 days.

Fun with Grape

Ingredients:

Grapes- 6 cup
Apple- 1 piece

Ginger- 2"
Blackberry- ½ cup
Broccoli- 2 cup
Spinach- 1 cup

Directions:

1. Blend everything for two-three minutes.
Enjoy

An easy one

Ingredients:

Melon- ½ cup
Pineapple- ½ cup
Apple- 1 piece
Spinach- 1 handful

Directions:

1. Blend everything for two-three minutes.
Enjoy

An workout smoothie

Ingredients:

Pear- 1 piece
Peach- 1 piece
Apricots- 2 piece
Water- 1 cup
Spinach- 1 handful

Directions:

1. Blend everything for two-three minutes.
Enjoy

Green Orange Smoothie

Ingredients:

Orange- 1 piece

Broccoli- 1 cup
Kiwi- 1 piece

Directions:

1. Blend everything for two-three minutes.
Enjoy

A Common Smoothie

Ingredients:

Figs- 4
Water- 1 cup
Banana- 1 piece
Milk- 1 cup
Flax seed- 1tsp
Protein powder- 1 tsp.

Directions:

1. Blend everything for two-three minutes.
Enjoy

Another Work out Smoothie

Ingredients:

Cantaloape- ¼ piece
Pineapple- ¼ piece
Guava- 2 piece
Broccoli- 1 cup

Directions:

1. Blend everything for two-three minutes.
Enjoy

Easy to Pick Smoothie

Ingredients:

Tomato- 1 piece
Cabbage- 1/3 cups

Packed Parsley- 1 cup
Celery- 2 stalks
Spinach- 2 cups

Directions:

1. Blend everything for two-three minutes.
Enjoy

Go for it Smoothie

Ingredients:

Tomatoes- 4 piece
Cucumber- 1 piece
Celery- 2 stalks
Bell pepper- 1 piece
Onion- 1/4th piece
Parsley leaves- 2 cups
Lime- 1 piece

Directions:

1. Blend everything for two-three minutes.
Enjoy

Smoothie of Sunset

Ingredients:

Potato- 1 piece
Carrot- 1 piece
Pepper- 1 piece
Red Beets- 2 piece
Apples- 2 piece
Orange- 1 piece
Spinach- 2 cup

Directions:

1. Blend everything for two-three minutes.
Enjoy

Plumber Beet

Ingredients:

Kale- 2 cups
Coconut water- 2 cups
Raspberry- 2 cups
Plum- 1 large
Beet- ½ piece

Directions:

1. Blend everything for two-three minutes.
Enjoy

Fun with Raspberry

Ingredients:

Kale- 2 cups
Coconut water- 2 cups
Raspberry- 2 cups
Apple- 1 piece

Directions:

1. Blend everything for two-three minutes.
Enjoy

Orchard of Summer

Ingredients:

Spinach- 2 cups
Water- 2 cups
Peach- 1 piece
Plum- 1 large
Apricots- 2 piece

Directions:

1. Blend everything for two-three minutes.
Enjoy

Pear apple fun

Ingredients:

Pears- 2 piece
Apples- 2 piece
Beets- 2 piece
Carrot- 1 piece
Cabbage- 1 cup
Chard- 2 cup
Kale- 2 cup
Spinach- 1 cup

Directions:

1. Blend everything for two-three minutes.
Enjoy

Kiwi with Berry

Ingredients:

Pineapple- ¼ large
Blackberry- 1 cup
Spinach- 2 cups
Kiwi- 1 piece
Pear- 1/4th piece
Coconut water- ¼ cup
Mint- 30 leaves

Directions:

1. Pour everything at once in blender
2. Blend for at least 3 minutes.
Enjoy

Pie of Apple

Ingredients:

Butternut squash- 4 cups
Honeycrisp apple- 1 piece
Cinnamon- 2 cup
Spinach- 2 cup

Directions:

1. Pour everything at once in blender
2. Blend for at least 3 minutes.

Enjoy

Goody Good Smoothie

Ingredients:

Beets- 2 cup
Carrot- 2 cup
Strawberry- 1 cup
Kale- 2 cups

Directions:

1. Pour everything at once in blender
2. Blend for at least 3 minutes.

Enjoy

Goodness Smoothie

Ingredients:

Kale- 2 cups
Apple- 1 piece
Pear- ½ piece
Strawberry- 10 piece
Water- 1 cup

Directions:

1. Pour everything at once in blender
2. Blend for at least 3 minutes.

Enjoy

Mean Greeny Juice

Ingredients:

Celery- 3 stalks
Cucumbers- 2 piece

Spinach- 5 fresh leaves
Parsley- ½ cup
Wheat grass- 3 inch
Water- 2 cup

Directions:

1. Pour everything at once in blender
2. Blend for at least 3 minutes.
Enjoy

Veggy Smoothie

Ingredients:

Celery- 3 stalks
Carrots- 2 piece
Red Beet- ½ piece
Spinach- 5 leaves
Alfalfa sprouts- ½ cup
Wheat grass- 3 inch
Water- 2 cups

Directions:

1. Pour everything at once in blender
2. Blend for at least 3 minutes.
Enjoy

Grass of Apple

Ingredients:

Apples- 3 piece
Wheat grass- 3 inch
Water- 2 cups

Directions:

1. Pour everything at once in blender
2. Blend for at least 3 minutes.
Enjoy

Grass of Wheat

Ingredients:

Oranges- 2 pieces
Banana- 1 piece
Berry- ½ cup
Wheat Grass- 2 inch
Ice Cubes- 1 cup

Directions:

1. Pour everything at once in blender
2. Blend for at least 3 minutes.

Enjoy

Grass of Orange

Ingredients:

Orange- 2 piece
Carrots- 2 piece
Wheat Grass- 3inch

Directions:

1. Pour everything at once in blender
2. Blend for at least 3 minutes.

Enjoy

Winter green smoothie

Ingredients:

Apples- 4 piece
Pears- 2 piece
Celery- 2 sticks
Kale- large bunch
Watercress- 1 small bunch
Chili- 1 small size

Directions:

1. Pour everything at once in blender
2. Blend for at least 3 minutes.

Enjoy

Spring with Green Smoothie

Ingredients:

Lettuce- 2 heads
Spring greens- 4 cups
Cucumber- 1 piece
Sprig of parsley- 1 small piece
Lemon juice- 1 piece

Directions:

1. Pour everything at once in blender
2. Blend for at least 3 minutes.

Enjoy

Summer with Green Smoothie

Ingredients:

cucumber- ½ piece
Honeydew melon- ½ piece
Seedless grapes- small bunch
kiwi- 2 pieces
Spinach- 2 cup
Mint- 1 small cup
Lemon juice- ½ cup

Directions:

1. Pour everything at once in blender
2. Blend for at least 3 minutes.

Enjoy

Fall in love Smoothie

Ingredients:

Apples- 3 pieces
Cucumber- 1 piece
Celery- 3 sticks
Grapes- small bunch
Honeydew- 1 large pice
Basil- small sprig

Directions:

1. Pour everything at once in blender
2. Blend for at least 3 minutes.
Enjoy

Carrot with Spinach

Ingredients:

Carrots- 5 piece
Spinach- 1 cup

Directions:

1. Pour everything at once in blender
2. Blend for at least 3 minutes.
Enjoy

Raw Spinach Fun Smoothie

Ingredients:

Spinach- 1 bunch
Raw honey- 1 teaspoon

Directions:

1. Pour everything at once in blender
2. Blend for at least 3 minutes.
Enjoy

Spinach with Tomato

Ingredients:

Spinach- 1 cup
Tomato- 4 pieces

Directions:

1. Pour everything at once in blender
2. Blend for at least 3 minutes.
Enjoy

Spinach with Beet Carrot

Ingredients:

Beet- ½ with top
Carrot- 3 piece
Spinach- ½ cup

Directions:

1. Pour everything at once in blender
2. Blend for at least 3 minutes.
Enjoy

Cucumber and Spinach mix

Ingredients:

carrots- 4 pieces
apple- 1 piece
Cucumber- ¼ piece
Spinach- 1 cup

Directions:

1. Pour everything at once in blender
2. Blend for at least 3 minutes.
Enjoy

An smoothie full of Calcium

Ingredients:

Broccoli- ½ cup
Carrot- 3 piece
Apple- 1 piece
Fresh parsley- 1 dash
Lemon- ½ piece

Directions:

1. Pour everything at once in blender
2. Blend for at least 3 minutes.
Enjoy

Cale Smoothie

Ingredients:

Apple- 1 piece
Kale- 3 piece
Celery- 1 cup

Directions:

1. Pour everything at once in blender
2. Blend for at least 3 minutes.
Enjoy

Weight loss help smoothie

Ingredients:

Jerusalem artichoke- 1 piece
Carrots- 4 piece
Beet- ½ piece
Spinach- 2 cups

Directions:

1. Pour everything at once in blender
2. Blend for at least 3 minutes.

Enjoy

Fun with Berry

Ingredients:

Grapefruit- 1 piece
Strawberry- 8 piece
Orange- 1 piece
Lemon- ½ piece
Spinach- 2 handful

Directions:

1. Pour everything at once in blender
2. Blend for at least 3 minutes.

Enjoy

Berry with apple

Ingredients:

Apples- 2 piece
Strawberry- 1 cup
Raspberry- ½ cup
Spinach- 1 cup

Directions:

1. Pour everything at once in blender
2. Blend for at least 3 minutes.

Enjoy

Berry with Water

Ingredients:

Watermelon- 1/4th piece
strawberry- 1 cup
Blueberry- 1 cup
Lemon- 1 piece
Spinach- 2 cup

Directions:

1. Pour everything at once in blender
2. Blend for at least 3 minutes.
Enjoy

Greeny Lemonade cum Smoothie

Ingredients:

Romaine lettuce- 8 leaves
Apples- 2 piece
Lemon- 2 piece
Carrot- 1 piece

Directions:

1. Pour everything at once in blender
2. Blend for at least 3 minutes.
Enjoy

Honey green smoothie

Ingredients:

Honeydew melon- ¼ piece
Fresh mint- 3stalks
Lime wedge- 1 piece

Directions:

1. Pour everything at once in blender
2. Blend for at least 3 minutes.
Enjoy

Lemon Fun

Ingredients:

Blackberry- 1 cup
Lemon- ½ cup
Apple- 1 piece
Ice Cubes- ½ cup

Water- 1 cup

Directions:

1. Pour everything at once in blender
2. Blend for at least 3 minutes.

Enjoy

Low Blood Sugar Magic

Ingredients:

Beetroot- 1 piece
Cucumber- 1 piece
Corn- 1 piece
Potato- 1 piece
Tomato- 1 piece
Blueberry- ½ cup
Lemon- 1 piece
spinach- 1 cup

Directions:

1. Pour everything at once in blender
2. Blend for at least 3 minutes.

Enjoy

Soy smoothie

Ingredients:

Banana- 1 piece
Strawberry- ½ cup
Raspberry- ½ cup
Cherry- ½ cup
Soy milk- 1 cup
Soy yogurt- ½ cup
Spinach- 1 cup

Directions:

1. Pour everything at once in blender
2. Blend for at least 3 minutes.

Enjoy

Ice Smoothie

Ingredients:

Strawberry- ½ cup
Banana- 1 piece
Peach- 1 large
Soy milk- ½ cup
Soy ice-cream- ½ cup
Spinach- 2 cup

Directions:

1. Pour everything at once in blender
2. Blend for at least 3 minutes.
Enjoy

Mixed Green Smoothie

Ingredients:

banana- 2 piece
Spinach- 2 huge handful
Almond milk- 1 cup
Cinnamon- ¼ teaspoon
Coconut oil- 1 table spoon

Directions:

1. Pour everything at once in blender
2. Blend for at least 3 minutes.
Enjoy

Mango Smoothie

Ingredients:

Spinach- 2 cup
Mango- 1 piece
Banana- 1 piece
Pineapple- 1 cup

Water- 1 cup

Directions:

1. Pour everything at once in blender
2. Blend for at least 3 minutes.
Enjoy

Popsicle Green Smoothie

Ingredients:

Spinach- 2 cups
Frozen berry- 2 cups
Banana- 2 piece
Water- 1 cup

Directions:

1. Pour everything at once in blender
2. Blend for at least 3 minutes.
Enjoy

Julius Smoothie

Ingredients:

Orange juice- ½ cup
Mango- 2 piece
Spinach/Parsley- 2 cups
Ice- 2 cups
Honey- 1 tea spoon

Directions:

1. Put everything in your blender and turn it on.
2. Blend for four minutes.
Enjoy

Ginger Smoothie

Ingredients:

Organic berry- 1 cup
Spinach- 2 cups
Water- 2 cups
Ginger root- ¼ inch

Directions:

1. Put everything in your blender and turn it on.
2. Blend for four minutes.

Enjoy

Aloe vera Smoothie

Ingredients:

Liquid aloe vera- ½ cup
Blueberry- 1 cup
Raspberry- 1 cup
Soy protein- 1 scoop
Celery- 1 piece
Cucumber- ½ piece

Directions:

1. Put everything in your blender and turn it on.
2. Blend for four minutes.

Enjoy

Smoothie of Banana

Ingredients:

Banana- 2 piece
Vanilla yogurt- 1 cup
Milk- 1 cup
Honey- 2 tsp
Cinnamon- 1 pinch
Ice- 1 cup
Spinach- 2 cup

Directions:

1. Put everything in your blender and turn it on.
2. Blend for four minutes.

Enjoy

The Directions will be same for following Smoothies. Here that is:

1. You have to take all the ingredients and you have to wash them properly.
2. Then simply add everything to your blender at once
3. Blend for 3-4 minutes.
4. Take it out and use ice cubes to make it cold.

Enjoy

Strawberry with Banana mix smoothie

Ingredients:

Banana- 1 piece
Strawberry- 1 cup
Vanilla yogurt- ½ cup
Honey- 1 tea spoon
Cinnamon- 1 pinch
Broccoli- 2 cups

The Directions will be same for following Smoothies. Here that is:

1. You have to take all the ingredients and you have to wash them properly.
2. Then simply add everything to your blender at once
3. Blend for 3-4 minutes.
4. Take it out and use ice cubes to make it cold.

Enjoy

Berry Fun Smoothie

Ingredients:

Blackberry- ½ cup
Strawberry- ½ cup
Raspberry- ½ cup
Milk- 1 cup
Ice- 1 cup
Spinach- 1 cup

The Directions will be same for following Smoothies. Here that is:

1. You have to take all the ingredients and you have to wash them properly.
2. Then simply add everything to your blender at once
3. Blend for 3-4 minutes.
4. Take it out and use ice cubes to make it cold.

Enjoy

Straw-Bana peach

Ingredients:

Kale- 2 cups
Water- 1 cup
Orange- 1 piece
Peach- 1 piece
Strawberry- 1 cup
Banana- 1 piece

The Directions will be same for following Smoothies. Here that is:

1. You have to take all the ingredients and you have to wash them properly.
2. Then simply add everything to your blender at once
3. Blend for 3-4 minutes.
4. Take it out and use ice cubes to make it cold.

Enjoy

Arugula Smoothie

Ingredients:

Milk- 1 cup
Arugula- ½ cup
Baby spinach- ½ cup
Blueberry- ½ cup
Chia seeds- 1 tablespoon
Coconut oil- 1 tablespoon
Sea salt- 1 dash
Honey- 1 tablespoon

The Directions will be same for following Smoothies. Here that is:

1. You have to take all the ingredients and you have to wash them properly.
2. Then simply add everything to your blender at once

3. Blend for 3-4 minutes.
4. Take it out and use ice cubes to make it cold.

Enjoy

Arugula with Green Smoothie

Ingredients:

Water- 1 cup
Avocado- ½ cup
Arugula- ½ cup
Spinach- ½ cup
Blueberry- ½ cup
Cinnamon- ½ teaspoon
Honey- ½ tablespoon

The Directions will be same for following Smoothies. Here that is:
1. You have to take all the ingredients and you have to wash them properly.
2. Then simply add everything to your blender at once
3. Blend for 3-4 minutes.
4. Take it out and use ice cubes to make it cold.

Enjoy

Arugula Magic Smoothie

Ingredients:

Water- 1 cup
Arugula- ½ cup
Spinach- ½ cup
Banana- 1 cup
Strawberry- ½ cup
Coconut oil- 1 teaspoon
Sea salt- 1 dash
Blueberry- ½ cup
Raspberry- ½ cup

The Directions will be same for following Smoothies. Here that is:
1. You have to take all the ingredients and you have to wash them properly.
2. Then simply add everything to your blender at once
3. Blend for 3-4 minutes.

4. Take it out and use ice cubes to make it cold.
Enjoy

Banana Beet Smoothie

Ingredients:

Water- 1 cup
Beet greens- 1 cup
Banana- 1 piece
Chia seed- 1 tablespoon
Stevia- optional

The Directions will be same for following Smoothies. Here that is:
1. You have to take all the ingredients and you have to wash them properly.
2. Then simply add everything to your blender at once
3. Blend for 3-4 minutes.
4. Take it out and use ice cubes to make it cold.
Enjoy

Blueberry, apple and Beet Green Smoothie

Ingredients:

Apple- 1 piece
Blueberry- ½ cup
Banana- ½ piece
Beet green- 2 cups
Cinnamon- ½ teaspoon
Honey- optional

The Directions will be same for following Smoothies. Here that is:
1. You have to take all the ingredients and you have to wash them properly.
2. Then simply add everything to your blender at once
3. Blend for 3-4 minutes.
4. Take it out and use ice cubes to make it cold.
Enjoy

Detox of Spring Smoothie

Ingredients:

Water- 1 cup
Lemon- ½ cup
Kale leaves- 1 cup
Dandelion green- 1 cup
Apple- 1 cup
Pear- 1 cup
Ginger- ½ teaspoon
Cayenne pepper- ¼ teaspoon
Honey- optional

The Directions will be same for following Smoothies. Here that is:

1. You have to take all the ingredients and you have to wash them properly.
2. Then simply add everything to your blender at once
3. Blend for 3-4 minutes.
4. Take it out and use ice cubes to make it cold.

Enjoy

Dandelion Fun Smoothie

Ingredients:

Water- 1 cup
Dandelion green- 1 cup
Frozen banana- 1 piece
Strawberry- ½ cup
Blueberry- ½ cup
Honey- optional

The Directions will be same for following Smoothies. Here that is:

1. You have to take all the ingredients and you have to wash them properly.
2. Then simply add everything to your blender at once
3. Blend for 3-4 minutes.
4. Take it out and use ice cubes to make it cold.

Enjoy

Apple of Dandelion Smoothie

Ingredients:

Water- 1 cup
Apple- 1 piece
Banana- 1 piece
Dandelion green- 1 cup
Lemon- ½ cup

The Directions will be same for following Smoothies. Here that is:

1. You have to take all the ingredients and you have to wash them properly.
2. Then simply add everything to your blender at once
3. Blend for 3-4 minutes.
4. Take it out and use ice cubes to make it cold.

Enjoy

Watermelon Green Detox Smoothie

Ingredients:

Water- ½ cup
Watermelon- 1 cup
Banana- 1 piece
Dandelion green- 1 cup
Juice- ½ lime
Cinnamon- ½ teaspoon
Maple syrup- optional

The Directions will be same for following Smoothies. Here that is:

1. You have to take all the ingredients and you have to wash them properly.
2. Then simply add everything to your blender at once
3. Blend for 3-4 minutes.
4. Take it out and use ice cubes to make it cold.

Enjoy

Spicy green smoothie

Ingredients:

Water- 1 cup

Avocado- ½ piece
Baby Spinach- 1 cup
Kale- 1 cup
Blueberry- ½ cup
Chia Seed- 1 tsp
Coconut oil- ½ tsp
Chili powder- ¼ tsp
Honey- ½ tsp

The Directions will be same for following Smoothies. Here that is:

1. You have to take all the ingredients and you have to wash them properly.
2. Then simply add everything to your blender at once
3. Blend for 3-4 minutes.
4. Take it out and use ice cubes to make it cold.

Enjoy

Kale Smoothie

Ingredients:

Kombucha- 1 cup
Kale- 1 cup
Avocado- ½ cup
Blueberry/Raspberry/Pineapple/Papaya- ½ cup
Coconut oil- 1 tablespoon
Cinnamon- 1 dash
Honey- optional

The Directions will be same for following Smoothies. Here that is:

1. You have to take all the ingredients and you have to wash them properly.
2. Then simply add everything to your blender at once
3. Blend for 3-4 minutes.
4. Take it out and use ice cubes to make it cold.

Enjoy

Energizer Smoothie

Ingredients:

Coconut water- 1 cup
Banana- 1 piece

Tropical fruit- ½ cup
Spinach- ½ cup
Kale- ½ cup
Greek yogurt- 1/3 cup
Goji berry- ¼ cup
Cranberry- ¼ cup
Coconut flakes- ¼ cup
Coconut oil- 1 tablespoon
Maca- 1 tablespoon
Wheat Grass- 1 tablespoon
Honey- optional

The Directions will be same for following Smoothies. Here that is:

1. You have to take all the ingredients and you have to wash them properly.
2. Then simply add everything to your blender at once
3. Blend for 3-4 minutes.
4. Take it out and use ice cubes to make it cold.

Enjoy

Mean detox green

Ingredients:

Water- 1 cup
Lemon juice- ½ cup
Banana- 1 piece
Kale- 1 cup
Spirulina- 1 teaspoon
Chlorella- 1 teaspoon
Celtic sea salt- 1 dash
Honey- 1 tablespoon
Ice cubes- 3-5 cubes

The Directions will be same for following Smoothies. Here that is:

1. You have to take all the ingredients and you have to wash them properly.
2. Then simply add everything to your blender at once
3. Blend for 3-4 minutes.
4. Take it out and use ice cubes to make it cold.

Enjoy

Killing Kale Smoothie

Ingredients:

Almond milk- 1 cup
Banana- 1 piece
Kale- 1 cup
Chia Seed- 1 tablespoon
Coconut oil- ½ tablespoon
Cinnamon- ¼ tablespoon
Honey- optional

The Directions will be same for following Smoothies. Here that is:

1. You have to take all the ingredients and you have to wash them properly.
2. Then simply add everything to your blender at once
3. Blend for 3-4 minutes.
4. Take it out and use ice cubes to make it cold.

Enjoy

Fun with Lettuce

Ingredients:

Water- 1 cup
Lettuce- 2 cup
Banana- 1 cup
Mixed berry- 1 cup
Flax seed- 1 tablespoon
Honey- optional

The Directions will be same for following Smoothies. Here that is:

1. You have to take all the ingredients and you have to wash them properly.
2. Then simply add everything to your blender at once
3. Blend for 3-4 minutes.
4. Take it out and use ice cubes to make it cold.

Enjoy

Tropical Lettuce Green

Ingredients:

Water- 1 cup
Romaine lettuce- 2 cup
Pineapples- ½ cup
Mango- ½ cup
Banana- ½ piece
Stevia- optional

Glowing green smoothie

Ingredients:

Water- 2 cups
Spinach- 6 cups
Romaine lettuce- 5 cups
Organic celery- 2 stalks
Organic apple- 1 piece
Pear- 1 piece
Banana- 1 piece
Lemon juice- 2 table spoon

The Directions will be same for following Smoothies. Here that is:
1. You have to take all the ingredients and you have to wash them properly.
2. Then simply add everything to your blender at once
3. Blend for 3-4 minutes.
4. Take it out and use ice cubes to make it cold.
Enjoy

Strawberry and Salad Smoothie

Ingredients:

Water- 1 cup
Fresh Salad- 1 cup
Banana- 1 piece
Strawberry- 1 cup
Coconut oil- 1 tsp
Sea salt- 1 dash
Honey- optional

The Directions will be same for following Smoothies. Here that is:

1. You have to take all the ingredients and you have to wash them properly.
2. Then simply add everything to your blender at once
3. Blend for 3-4 minutes.
4. Take it out and use ice cubes to make it cold.

Enjoy

Glow with Green Smoothie

Ingredients:

Water- 2 cups
Spinach- 6 cups
Lettuce- 5 cups
Celery- 2 stalks
Apple- 1 piece
193. Rosemary Smoothie

Ingredients:

Water- 1 cup
Banana- 1 piece
Baby Spinach- 1 cup
Blueberry- 1 cup
Rosemary- 1 sprig
Salt- 1 dash
Maple syrup- optional

The Directions will be same for following Smoothies. Here that is:

1. You have to take all the ingredients and you have to wash them properly.
2. Then simply add everything to your blender at once
3. Blend for 3-4 minutes.
4. Take it out and use ice cubes to make it cold.

Enjoy

Avocado Arugula Smoothie

Ingredients:

Water- 1 cup
Avocado- ½ piece
Arugula- ½ cup

Spinach- ½ cup
Blueberries- ½ cup
Cinnamon- ½ tsp
Honey- ½ tsp

The Directions will be same for following Smoothies. Here that is:
1. You have to take all the ingredients and you have to wash them properly.
2. Then simply add everything to your blender at once
3. Blend for 3-4 minutes.
4. Take it out and use ice cubes to make it cold.
Enjoy

Spirulina Smoothie

Ingredients:
Water- 1.5 cup
Banana- 1 piece
Spinach- 1 cup
Spirulina powder- 1 tsp
Cacao powder- 1 tsp
Celtic salt- 1 dash
Honey- optional
196. Aloe Smoothie Recipe

Ingredients:
Water- 1 cup
Aloe vera leaf- 1 piece
Spinach- 1 cup
Blueberry- ½ cup
Coconut oil- 1 tsp
Sea salt- 1 dash
Honey- optional

The Directions will be same for following Smoothies. Here that is:
1. You have to take all the ingredients and you have to wash them properly.
2. Then simply add everything to your blender at once
3. Blend for 3-4 minutes.
4. Take it out and use ice cubes to make it cold.
Enjoy

Spicy and fun Smoothie

Ingredients:

Water- 1 cup
Avocado- ½ medium
Baby spinach- 1 cup
Blueberry- ½ cup
Chia seeds- 1 tsp
Coconut oil- ½ tsp
Chili powder- ¼ tsp
honey- ½ tsp

The Directions will be same for following Smoothies. Here that is:

1. You have to take all the ingredients and you have to wash them properly.
2. Then simply add everything to your blender at once
3. Blend for 3-4 minutes.
4. Take it out and use ice cubes to make it cold.

Enjoy

Get your Energy Smoothie

Ingredients:

Coconut water- 1cup
Banana- 1 piece
Tropical fruit- ½ cup
Spinach- ½ cup
Kale- ½ cup
Greek yogurt- 1/3 cup
Cranberries- ¼ cup
Coconut flakes- ¼ cup
Maca- 1 tsp
Wheat grass powder- 1 tsp
Honey- optional

The Directions will be same for following Smoothies. Here that is:

1. You have to take all the ingredients and you have to wash them properly.
2. Then simply add everything to your blender at once
3. Blend for 3-4 minutes.
4. Take it out and use ice cubes to make it cold.

Enjoy

Basil Green Smoothie

Ingredients:

Water- 1 cup
Banana- 1 piece
Basil leaves- 8 piece
Berries- 1 cup
Coconut oil- 1 tablespoon
cinnamon- ¼ teaspoon
Stevia- optional
200. Arugula Smoothie

Ingredients:

Milk- 1 cup
Arugula- ½ cup
Baby spinach- ½ cup
Blueberry- ½ cup
Chia seed- 1 tablespoon
Coconut oil- 1 tablespoon
Sea salt- 1 dash
Honey- 1 tablespoon

The Directions will be same for following Smoothies. Here that is:

1. You have to take all the ingredients and you have to wash them properly.
2. Then simply add everything to your blender at once
3. Blend for 3-4 minutes.
4. Take it out and use ice cubes to make it cold.

Enjoy

Arugula smoothie

Ingredients:

Milk- 1 cup
Arugula- ½ cup
Baby spinach- ½ cup
Blueberry- ½ cup
Chia seed- 1 tablespoon
Coconut oil- 1 tablespoon

Honey- 1 tablespoon

The Directions will be same for following Smoothies. Here that is:
1. You have to take all the ingredients and you have to wash them properly.
2. Then simply add everything to your blender at once
3. Blend for 3-4 minutes.
4. Take it out and use ice cubes to make it cold.

Enjoy

Simple Banana Smoothie

Ingredients:

Almond milk- ½ cups
Banana- 1 piece
Spinach- 1 cup
Mango chunks- ½ cup
Greek yogurt- 2 tablespoon
Chia seeds- 1 tablespoon
Bee pollen- 1 teaspoon

The Directions will be same for following Smoothies. Here that is:
1. You have to take all the ingredients and you have to wash them properly.
2. Then simply add everything to your blender at once
3. Blend for 3-4 minutes.
4. Take it out and use ice cubes to make it cold.

Enjoy

Mango lime Smoothie

Ingredients:

Water- 1 cup
Avocado- ½ cup
Cilantro- ½ cup
Spinach- 1 cup
Mango chunks- 1 cup
Juice lime- 1 tsp
Ginger powder- ½ tablespoon
Raw honey- ½ tablespoon

The Directions will be same for following Smoothies. Here that is:

1. You have to take all the ingredients and you have to wash them properly.
2. Then simply add everything to your blender at once
3. Blend for 3-4 minutes.
4. Take it out and use ice cubes to make it cold.

Enjoy

Spinach with Ginger Fun

Ingredients:

Water- 1 cup
Baby spinach- 1 cup
Avocado- ½ cup
Banana- ½ piece
Blueberry- ½ cup
Ginger- 1/4th inch
Honey- ½ tsp

The Directions will be same for following Smoothies. Here that is:

1. You have to take all the ingredients and you have to wash them properly.
2. Then simply add everything to your blender at once
3. Blend for 3-4 minutes.
4. Take it out and use ice cubes to make it cold.

Enjoy

Superfood Smoothie

Ingredients:

Water- 1 cup
Banana- 1 piece
Blueberry- ½ cup
Spinach- 1 cup
Kale- ½ cup
Coconut oil- 1 tsp
Spirulina- 1 tsp
Cinnamon- ¼ tsp

The Directions will be same for following Smoothies. Here that is:

1. You have to take all the ingredients and you have to wash them properly.

2. Then simply add everything to your blender at once
3. Blend for 3-4 minutes.
4. Take it out and use ice cubes to make it cold.
Enjoy

Ginger Pear Smoothie

Ingredients:

Water- 1 cup
Pear- 1 medium piece
Baby spinach- 1 cup
Flax- 1 tsp
Coconut oil- 1 tsp
Ginger- ¼ inch
Honey- ½ tsp

The Directions will be same for following Smoothies. Here that is:
1. You have to take all the ingredients and you have to wash them properly.
2. Then simply add everything to your blender at once
3. Blend for 3-4 minutes.
4. Take it out and use ice cubes to make it cold.
Enjoy

Apple Green Smoothie

Ingredients:

Organic apple juice- 1 cup
Apple- 1 piece
Strawberry- ½ cup
Spinach- 1 cup
Coconut oil- 1 teaspoon
Cinnamon- ½ teaspoon

The Directions will be same for following Smoothies. Here that is:
1. You have to take all the ingredients and you have to wash them properly.
2. Then simply add everything to your blender at once
3. Blend for 3-4 minutes.
4. Take it out and use ice cubes to make it cold.

Enjoy

Ormus smoothie of Supergreen

Ingredients:

Almond milk- 1 cup
Banana- 1 piece
Spinach- 1 cup
Blueberry- ½ cup
Sun Warrior Supergreens- 1 tsp
Coconut oil- ½ tsp
Cinnamon- ¼ tsp
Vanilla powder- ¼ tsp
Himalayan Salt- 1 dash
Honey- optional

The Directions will be same for following Smoothies. Here that is:
1. You have to take all the ingredients and you have to wash them properly.
2. Then simply add everything to your blender at once
3. Blend for 3-4 minutes.
4. Take it out and use ice cubes to make it cold.
Enjoy

Spinach with Minty Flavor

Ingredients:

Almond milk- 1 cup
Frozen banana- 1 piece
Spinach- 1 cup
Mint Leaves- 1 tsp
Blueberry- 1 tsp
Maple syrup- optional

Green Tea Smoothie Fun

Ingredients:

Brewed Green Tea- 1 cup
Frozen Banana- 1 piece
Baby Spinach- 1 cup
Coconut Oil- 1 tsp

Honey- 1 tsp

The Directions will be same for following Smoothies. Here that is:
1. You have to take all the ingredients and you have to wash them properly.
2. Then simply add everything to your blender at once
3. Blend for 3-4 minutes.
4. Take it out and use ice cubes to make it cold.
Enjoy

Blueberry with Spinach fun

Ingredients:

Water- 1 cup
Spinach- 2 cups
Blueberry- ½ cup
Banana- 1 piece
Stevia- 1 tsp

The Directions will be same for following Smoothies. Here that is:
1. You have to take all the ingredients and you have to wash them properly.
2. Then simply add everything to your blender at once
3. Blend for 3-4 minutes.
4. Take it out and use ice cubes to make it cold.
Enjoy

Kiwi Banana Smoothie

Ingredients:

Water- ½ cup
Kiwis- 2 pieces
Banana- 1 piece
Spinach- 1 cup
Sea Salt- 1 dash
Honey- 1 tsp

The Directions will be same for following Smoothies. Here that is:
1. You have to take all the ingredients and you have to wash them properly.
2. Then simply add everything to your blender at once

3. Blend for 3-4 minutes.
4. Take it out and use ice cubes to make it cold.
Enjoy

Full of Iron Smoothie

Ingredients:

Almond milk- 1 cup
Spinach- 2 cups
Spirulina- 4 tsp
Ripened banana- 1 piece

Arugula Smoothie

Ingredients:

Water- 1 cup
Arugula- ½ cup
Spinach- ½ cup
Banana- 1 piece
Strawberry- ½ cup
coconut oil- 1 tsp
Sea salt- 1 dash
Honey- optional

The Directions will be same for following Smoothies. Here that is:
1. You have to take all the ingredients and you have to wash them properly.
2. Then simply add everything to your blender at once
3. Blend for 3-4 minutes.
4. Take it out and use ice cubes to make it cold.
Enjoy

A Green Machine

Ingredients:

Water- 1 cup
Spinach- 1 cup
Kale- 1 cup
Green apple- 1 piece
Coconut oil- 1 tsp

Ginger- 1/4th piece
Stevia- optional

The Directions will be same for following Smoothies. Here that is:

1. You have to take all the ingredients and you have to wash them properly.
2. Then simply add everything to your blender at once
3. Blend for 3-4 minutes.
4. Take it out and use ice cubes to make it cold.

Enjoy

Peeper Smoothie

Ingredients:

Water- 1 cup
Spinach- 1 cup
Banana- 1 piece
Coconut oil- ½ tsp
Cayenne pepper- ¼ tsp
Honey- optional

The Directions will be same for following Smoothies. Here that is:

1. You have to take all the ingredients and you have to wash them properly.
2. Then simply add everything to your blender at once
3. Blend for 3-4 minutes.
4. Take it out and use ice cubes to make it cold.

Enjoy

Simple fun with Green Smoothie

Ingredients:

Water- 1 cup
Banana- 1 piece
Spinach- 1 cup

The Directions will be same for following Smoothies. Here that is:

1. You have to take all the ingredients and you have to wash them properly.
2. Then simply add everything to your blender at once
3. Blend for 3-4 minutes.

4. Take it out and use ice cubes to make it cold.
Enjoy

Smoothie of Aloe Vera

Ingredients:

Coconut oil- 1 cup
Aloe Vera leaf- ½ cup
Blueberry- ½ cup
Frozen Mango- ½ cup
Coconut oil- ½ tsp
Basil- 1 handful
Stevia- optional

The Directions will be same for following Smoothies. Here that is:
1. You have to take all the ingredients and you have to wash them properly.
2. Then simply add everything to your blender at once
3. Blend for 3-4 minutes.
4. Take it out and use ice cubes to make it cold.
Enjoy

Smoothie of Skin

Ingredients:

Water- 1 cup
Aloe Vera leaf- 1 piece
Avocado- ¼ piece
Kiwi- 1 piece
Blueberry- ½ cup
Coconut oil- 1 tsp
Salt- 1 pinch
Honey- 1 tsp

The Directions will be same for following Smoothies. Here that is:
1. You have to take all the ingredients and you have to wash them properly.
2. Then simply add everything to your blender at once
3. Blend for 3-4 minutes.
4. Take it out and use ice cubes to make it cold.
Enjoy

Smoothie of Aloe

Ingredients:

Water- 1 cup
Aloe vera leaf- 1 medium piece
Spinach- 1 cup
Blueberry- ½ cup
Coconut oil- 1 tsp
Celtic Sea Salt- 1 dash
Stevia- optional

The Directions will be same for following Smoothies. Here that is:

1. You have to take all the ingredients and you have to wash them properly.
2. Then simply add everything to your blender at once
3. Blend for 3-4 minutes.
4. Take it out and use ice cubes to make it cold.

Enjoy

Strawberry Fun

Ingredients:

Almond Milk- 1 cup
Diced aloe gel- ½ cup
Strawberry- ½ cup
Banana- ½ piece
Ice cube- 5 piece
Honey- optional

The Directions will be same for following Smoothies. Here that is:

1. You have to take all the ingredients and you have to wash them properly.
2. Then simply add everything to your blender at once
3. Blend for 3-4 minutes.
4. Take it out and use ice cubes to make it cold.

Enjoy

Lemonade with Aloe Vera

Ingredients:

Water- 1 cup
Avocado- ½ piece
Aloe vera- 1 medium piece
Lemon- ½ piece
Lime- ½ piece
Coconut oil- 1 tsp
Celtic salt- 1 dash
Honey- 1tsp

The Directions will be same for following Smoothies. Here that is:

1. You have to take all the ingredients and you have to wash them properly.
2. Then simply add everything to your blender at once
3. Blend for 3-4 minutes.
4. Take it out and use ice cubes to make it cold.

Enjoy

Superfood Smoothie

Ingredients:

Water- 1 cup
Banana- 1 piece
Blueberry- ½ cup
Spinach- 1 cup
Kale- ½ cup
Coconut oil- 1 tsp
Spirulina- 1 tsp
Cinnamon- ¼ tsp
Maple syrup- optional

The Directions will be same for following Smoothies. Here that is:

1. You have to take all the ingredients and you have to wash them properly.
2. Then simply add everything to your blender at once
3. Blend for 3-4 minutes.
4. Take it out and use ice cubes to make it cold.

Enjoy

Mean Green Smoothie

Ingredients:

Water- 1 cup
Lemon juice- ½ cup
Banana- 1 piece
Kale- 1 cup
Spirulina- 1 tsp
Chlorella- 1 tsp
Celtic sea salt- 1dash
Ice cubes- 3-5 piece

The Directions will be same for following Smoothies. Here that is:

1. You have to take all the ingredients and you have to wash them properly.
2. Then simply add everything to your blender at once
3. Blend for 3-4 minutes.
4. Take it out and use ice cubes to make it cold.

Enjoy

Basil Smoothie with Strawberry

Ingredients:

Water- 1 cup
Frozen Banana- 1 piece
Strawberry- ½ cup
Basil Leaves- 10 piece
Ice cubes- 6 piece
Stevia- optional

The Directions will be same for following Smoothies. Here that is:

1. You have to take all the ingredients and you have to wash them properly.
2. Then simply add everything to your blender at once
3. Blend for 3-4 minutes.
4. Take it out and use ice cubes to make it cold.

Enjoy

Basil Berry Smoothie

Ingredients:

Water- 1 cup
Banana- 1 piece
Spinach- 1 cup
Basil Leaves- 8 pieces
Frozen berries- 1 cup
Coconut oil- 1 tsp
Cinnamon- ¼ tsp
Stevia- optional

The Directions will be same for following Smoothies. Here that is:
1. You have to take all the ingredients and you have to wash them properly.
2. Then simply add everything to your blender at once
3. Blend for 3-4 minutes.
4. Take it out and use ice cubes to make it cold.
Enjoy

Awesome fun with Aloe Vera

Ingredients:

Coconut milk- 1 cup
Aloe Vera- 1 cup
Blueberry- ½ cup
Mango chunks- ½ cup
Coconut oil- ½ tsp
Basil- 1 handful
Stevia- optional

The Directions will be same for following Smoothies. Here that is:
1. You have to take all the ingredients and you have to wash them properly.
2. Then simply add everything to your blender at once
3. Blend for 3-4 minutes.
4. Take it out and use ice cubes to make it cold.
Enjoy

Cilantro of Tropical Smoothie

Ingredients:

Water- 1 cup

Cilantro- ½ cup
Pineapple- 1 cup
Mango- 1 cup
Lime juice- ½ cup
Celtic sea salt- 1 dash

The Directions will be same for following Smoothies. Here that is:

1. You have to take all the ingredients and you have to wash them properly.
2. Then simply add everything to your blender at once
3. Blend for 3-4 minutes.
4. Take it out and use ice cubes to make it cold.

Enjoy

Smoothie of Cilantro Recipe

Ingredients:

Water- 1 cup
Banana- 1 piece
Cilantro- ½ cup
Lime juice- ½ cup
Celtic sea salt- 1 dash
Honey- 1 dash

The Directions will be same for following Smoothies. Here that is:

1. You have to take all the ingredients and you have to wash them properly.
2. Then simply add everything to your blender at once
3. Blend for 3-4 minutes.
4. Take it out and use ice cubes to make it cold.

Enjoy

Green Smoothie of Guacamole

Ingredients:

Water- ½ cup
Avocado- 1 piece
Tomato- ½ cup
Cilantro- ¼ cup
Lime juice- ½ cup
Celtic sea salt- 1 dash

The Directions will be same for following Smoothies. Here that is:

1. You have to take all the ingredients and you have to wash them properly.
2. Then simply add everything to your blender at once
3. Blend for 3-4 minutes.
4. Take it out and use ice cubes to make it cold.

Enjoy

Mango Lime of Cilantro Smoothie

Ingredients:

Water- 1 cup
Avocado- ½ piece
Cilantro- ½ cup
Spinach- 1 cup
Mango chunks- 1 cup
Lime juice- 1 cup
Ginger powder- ½ teaspoon
Raw honey- ½ tablespoon

The Directions will be same for following Smoothies. Here that is:

1. You have to take all the ingredients and you have to wash them properly.
2. Then simply add everything to your blender at once
3. Blend for 3-4 minutes.
4. Take it out and use ice cubes to make it cold.

Enjoy

Fun with Banana Smoothie

Ingredients:

Almond Milk- 1.5 cup
Frozen Banana- 1 piece
Spinach- 1 cup
Mango chunks- ½ cup
Strawberries- ½ cup
Greek yogurt- 2tsp
Coconut oil- 1tsp
Chia seeds- 1tsp
Bee pollen- 1tsp

The Directions will be same for following Smoothies. Here that is:

1. You have to take all the ingredients and you have to wash them properly.
2. Then simply add everything to your blender at once
3. Blend for 3-4 minutes.
4. Take it out and use ice cubes to make it cold.

Enjoy

Kiwi with Banana Green Smoothie

Ingredients:

Water- ½ cup
Kiwis- 2 pieces
Banana- 1 fresh
Spinach- 1 cup
Sea Salt- 1 dash
Honey- optional

The Directions will be same for following Smoothies. Here that is:

1. You have to take all the ingredients and you have to wash them properly.
2. Then simply add everything to your blender at once
3. Blend for 3-4 minutes.
4. Take it out and use ice cubes to make it cold.

Enjoy

Skin Glow Smoothie

Ingredients:

Apple- 1 large
Cucumber- 1 medium size
Papaya- 1 piece
Celery- 6 stalks
Lemon- ½ piece
Ginger root- 1 piece

The Directions will be same for following Smoothies. Here that is:

1. You have to take all the ingredients and you have to wash them properly.
2. Then simply add everything to your blender at once
3. Blend for 3-4 minutes.

4. Take it out and use ice cubes to make it cold.

Enjoy

A glass of Sugarless Green Smoothie

Ingredients:

Apples- 3 pieces
Lemon- 1 piece
Ginger root- 1 piece
236. Spring Fun Smoothie

Ingredients:

Water- 1.5 cups
Lemon juice- ½ cup
Kale leaves- 1 cup
Dandelion green- 1 cup
Apple- 1 piece
Pear- 1 piece
Ginger- ½ teaspoon
Cayenne pepper- ¼ teaspoon
Honey- optional

The Directions will be same for following Smoothies. Here that is:

1. You have to take all the ingredients and you have to wash them properly.
2. Then simply add everything to your blender at once
3. Blend for 3-4 minutes.
4. Take it out and use ice cubes to make it cold.

Enjoy

Aloe Vera Lemon fun

Ingredients:

Water- 1 cup
Avocado- ½ piece
Aloe vera leaf- 1 medium piece
Lemon- ½ medium
Lime- ½ medium
Coconut oil- 1tsp
Celtic salt- 1 dash
Honey- 1 tsp

The Directions will be same for following Smoothies. Here that is:
1. You have to take all the ingredients and you have to wash them properly.
2. Then simply add everything to your blender at once
3. Blend for 3-4 minutes.
4. Take it out and use ice cubes to make it cold.
Enjoy

Beet with Berry

Ingredients:

Water- 1 cu[
Beet green- ½ cup
Cooked beet- ½ cup
Frozen blackberry- ½ cup
Frozen raspberry- ½ cup
Lemon- ½ piece
Coconut oil- 1tsp
Ginger- ¼ inch

The Directions will be same for following Smoothies. Here that is:
1. You have to take all the ingredients and you have to wash them properly.
2. Then simply add everything to your blender at once
3. Blend for 3-4 minutes.
4. Take it out and use ice cubes to make it cold.
Enjoy

Citrus Fun Smoothie

Ingredients:

Water- ½ cup
Orange- 1 piece
Lemon- 1 piece
Sea salt- 1 dash
Honey- 1tsp

The Directions will be same for following Smoothies. Here that is:
1. You have to take all the ingredients and you have to wash them properly.
2. Then simply add everything to your blender at once

3. Blend for 3-4 minutes.
4. Take it out and use ice cubes to make it cold.

Enjoy

Spinach juice

Ingredients:

5 stalks of spinach
3 apples
1 lemon
1 cucumber

Directions:

1. First of all clean all the ingredients with water.
2. Now take your blender, turn it on and add all the ingredients there.
3. If you are using a slow blender then you can add a little water in the blender.
4. Pour this healthy juice in your mug and enjoy.
5. Wash your blender properly when you are done.

Veggie green juice

Ingredients:

1 cup of fresh broccoli
1 cup cucumber
2 cup lettuce
½ green apple(you can skip this if you want)
1lime

Directions:

1. Wash your blender first.
2. Now simply add all the ingredients in the blender and turn it on.
3. It's better if you remove the pits of broccoli.
4. That is it.

Enjoy.

Lungs cleanser juice

Ingredients:

Kale- 3 leaves
1 large carrot
Celery- 3 stalks
1 inch slice ginger
Around ½ cup radish
1 lime

Directions:

1. Firstly, you need to remove the stems from the kale and the lime needs to be peeled properly.

2. Now add all this ingredients into your blender.

3. If you think the juice is very thick then add a little water.

4. To get the highest potency of this juice drink this within 15 minutes. If you want to store it then make sure that you store the juice in air tight jar in the freeze.

5. But don't keep the juice in the freeze more than one day.

Go green

Ingredients:

Romanie -5/6 leaves
¼ bunch of cilantro
½ lime
½ cup pineapple

Directions:

1. Switch on your blender and then put all the items in the blender.

2. Add the pineapple in the last.

3. You can make this juice cold by using frozen pineapples.

4. Serve it in your favorite mug.

Kiwi juice

Ingredients:

Kiwi fruits- 8 piece

3 fresh green apple
½ cucumber
About 2 inches of fresh ginger
Some fresh mint leave- 1 handful

Directions:

1. First of all, wash the kiwis, cucumber and apples with clean water
2. Now take your blender and put all the ingredients there.
3. Don't mix any extra sugar or anything.
4. Wait for 1 to 2 minutes to get the fresh juice.
5. Use ice cubes for serving.
6. Don't freeze this juice serve it immediately.

All about green

Ingredients:

½ cup of spinach
1 large garden fresh cucumber
1 large green apple
Celery-2 stalks
Parsley-3
1 tsp. of lemon juice
1 tsp. fresh ginger

Directions:

1. To make this juice first squeeze some lemons to get the lemon juice. As you need vey little amount of lemon juice so you don't need more than one lemon.
2. Now add all the ingredients with the lemon juice in the blender.
3. Use the ingredients frozen if you want the juice cold.
Enjoy.

Liver detox green juice

Ingredients:

½ cup green dandelions
½ cup parsley
1 lemon
½ rib celery
2 oranges

Directions:

1. First peeled out the oranges and lemon properly.
2. Now simply place all these ingredients in your blender.
3. It may take 1 or 2 minutes to get the fresh juice. In this juice you can also add the beet root for more nutrition.
4. Serve it with some mint leaves.

Enjoy.

Sweet Green

Ingredients:

beet root
3 kale leaves
4 lettuce leaves
Some spinach leaves
½ lemon
2 apples

Directions:

1. First of all, take out your blender and make sure that it is clean.
2. Now you need to remove the stems from the kale and also peel out the beet root.
3. When you have done with this add all the ingredients into your blender.
4. Use some ice cubes if you want it cool.
5. Serve and enjoy.

Tomato and radish juice

Ingredients:

2 tomatoes
4 parsley
½ lemon
2 radishes
2 lettuce leaves

Directions:

1. The making Directions is very simple for this juice. All you need to place all the ingredients in your blender.

2. Make sure that you have cleaned all the ingredients properly before putting them into the mixer.
3. Serve the juice with a lemon slice.

Enjoy.

Detox with cucumber and apple

Ingredients:

Fennel- 2 stalks
½ of a cucumber
½ fresh large green apple
Some mint leaves
1 inch of ginger root

Directions:

1. Turn on your blender on.
2. The ginger should be peeled properly.
3. Place all the ingredients in the blender and wait for 2 minutes.
4. Pour the juice in a mug.
5. Serve with some extra 2 /3 mint leaves.

Goodness of cabbage

Ingredients:

Green cabbage- 1 quarter head
Carrots-3
4 celery stalks

Directions:

1. You need to take a fresh cabbage otherwise the juice will not taste well.
2. Switch on your blender and place all the ingredients.
3. Use a low speed of your mixer.
4. You can add a little amount of water if you think the juice is very thick.

Enjoy.

Asparagus juice

Ingredients:

1 tomato
1 asparagus
1 cucumber
½ lemon

Directions:

1. In this juice the asparagus is the main ingredient, so first only take out the juice of the asparagus.
2. After that add the cucumber, tomato and lemon in the blender. Take out the juice and mic it with the asparagus juice.
3. Serve it immediately to get the best result.

Cleanse with dandelion

Ingredients:

1 handful of dandelion
Carrots -3/4
½ of a cucumber
½ lemon

Directions:

1. If you don't have dandelion then for this juice you can similarly use dandelion tincture.
2. You need to peel the lemon nicely.
3. Now turn on your blender and place all the ingredients.
4. And your juice is ready.

The boost up juice

Ingredients:

Apple -1
Kiwi-2
1 lime
Some spinach
1 stalk of celery
1 tsp. of fresh honey

Directions:

1. To start with this recipe first takes out the juice from lime. You can use your hands for this.
2. The kiwi needs to be peeled out nicely.
3. Okay now switch on your blender. Make sure that your blender is clean enough.
4. Now put all the ingredients in the blender.
5. Pour the juice in a mug and serve with some ice cubes.
6. It is better to drink it within 24-48 hours.

The ultimate green juice

Ingredients:

Spinach leaves –around 10 to 12
1 stalk celery
½ of a cucumber
½ cup parsley

Directions:

1. First of all wash all the vegetables with water.
2. Now simply put all the ingredients in your blender at once and use a medium speed of your blender.
3. Pour the juice in a mug.
4. You don't need to add any extra water as the cucumber will release a great amount of juice while juicing.
5. Serve with some mint leaves.

Enjoy.

Tropical green juice

Ingredients:

1 cup mango
1 cup pineapple chunks
½ cup coconut water
1 cup of baby spinach
½ cup of lime juice
¼ tsp. cayenne pepper

Directions:

1. To make this juice cold you can use frozen mangoes and pineapples.
2. make sure that you are using unsweetened coconut water for this juice.
3. If you don't have or don't want to use spinach then you can use any other leafy green like kale or collard green.
4. Firstly take out some juice from the lime.
5. Now switch on your blender and add all the ingredients there.
6. Pour the drink into two glasses.

Enjoy.

Green morning

Ingredients:

Romaine leaves -2
2 handful of spinach(or other green leaf)
1 Pomegranate
2 stalk of celery
Around 1 cup of blueberries
2/3 strawberries
1 cucumber
1 lemon
1 orange
½ of an apple

Directions:

1. For this juice you will need ¼ cup of pomegranate juice so first make this. You can use your blender for this.
2. Squeeze a lemon and use ¼ of the lemon juice.
3. Now switch on your blender and place all these.
4. Pour the juice into a mug and enjoy.
5. Try this juice in every morning.

Feel the green

Ingredients:

1 cucumber
2 large leaves of kale
1 cup spinach

2 large leaves of romaine lettuce
4 celery stalks
1 cup of coconut water.

Directions:

1. First of all, take your cutting board and cut the cucumber into 1 -2 inch pieces.
2. Cut the celery, spinach into smaller pieces and then add all the ingredients in your juicing bar.
3. Don't add the coconut water in the blender.
4. After you get the juice pour it into a mug and now mix the coconut water in the juice.
5. Make sure that you are using fresh and good organic coconut water.

Enjoy your juice.

Sweet broccoli juice

Ingredients:

3 heads of fresh broccoli
1/3 head cauliflower
½ red cabbage
3 carrots
2 tsp. of honey

Directions:

1. Take your blender and read out all the Directions carefully before you start juicing
2. Place all the ingredients in the blender.
3. Wait some time to get the juice.
4. Serve with ice cubes and enjoy.

Simple broccoli juice

Ingredients:

1 large broccoli
1 stalk celery
4 carrots
1 green apple

Directions:

1. First cut out the roots of the broccoli and clean all the ingredients properly.
2. Now turn on your blender and place all the ingredients there.
3. Wait until you get the juice.
4. Serve and enjoy.

Broccoli Synergy

Ingredients:

2 large heads of broccoli
3 cups nicely chopped broccoli Raab
6 carrots
3 apples
½ cups chopped fennel
2 inch ginger

Directions:

1. If you don't have broccoli Raab then you can easily skip this item. This only adds more sharp flavour in the juice.
2. Chopped the carrots and apples nicely so it can fit into your blender.
3. Now switch on your blender and simply put all the ingredients there. You will get around 32 ounces of juice by this.
4. Serve with ice cubes and enjoy.

Avocado juice

Ingredients:

½ large pineapple
6 cups chopped broccoli
6 kale
1 handful spinach
1 large cucumber
4 celery stalks
A little amount of ginger
1 avocado

Directions:

1. To make this yummy juice first you need to core and peel out the pineapple.

2. Cut the pineapple, cucumber and avocado so you can easily place them in the blender.

3. If you can't add all the ingredients in your blender at once then you can take out only the avocado juice from your blender. For that put the avocado in your blender.

4. After that when you have juiced the avocado put other ingredients in your blender and blends them.

5. Now transfer the avocado juice in the blender and blend one more time.

6. Serve immediately and enjoy.

Any time fruit juice

Ingredients:

1/3 of pineapple
½ of a cucumber
1 handful spinach
2 fresh green apples
2 limes

Directions:

1. To make this simple and easy juice you first need to the juice the lime separately. Pour the lime juice in your collection mug.

2. Now clean all the other ingredients properly and then place them in the blender.

3. Pour the juice in a mug with the lime juice.

4. Clean your blender.

Celery and carrot juice

Ingredients:

3 stalks of celery
1 ounce of parsley
3 medium size of carrots
1 large cucumber

Directions:

1. First cut the carrots and cucumber into small cubes so that it can fit into your blender.

2. Now take your blender and place all the ingredients there and start juicing.

3. Pour in a mug with some ice cubes.

4. To give some extra flavour adds an inch of ginger in the juice.
Enjoy.

Spinach and beet juice

Ingredients:

1 beet root
2 stalk large celery
3 cup spinach
Dried spirulina-1 tsp.

Directions:

1. Take your blender and read the Directions carefully before you start juicing.
2. Now simply add all the ingredients in the blender.
3. Take your mug and collect the juice from the blender.
4. Use some ice cubes if needed and enjoy.

Pure Kale juice

Ingredients:

1 medium size green apple
3 carrots
1 handful fresh cilantro
1 cup collard greens
4 leaf kale
1 medium pepper

Directions:

1. Cut the apples into cubes. Also cut the carrots so it can easily fit through your blender.
2. If you don't want to make the juice spicy then don't add pepper.
3. Make sure that you are using fresh cilantro.
4. Now take your blender and add all the ingredients there,
5. Serve with 1 or 2 leaf of parsley and enjoy.

Full of green

Ingredients:

3 medium size green apple
3 stalk celery
½ of a cucumber
4 leaf of kale
1 lemon
1 orange

Directions:

1. Clean all the ingredients with water first.
2. Squeeze the lemon properly and make sure you have peeled the orange.
3. Now put all the ingredients in blender and turn on your blender.
4. Pour the juice into a glass and serve.
5. Serve with a slice of a lemon.

Kale and orange juice

Ingredients:

6 leaves of kale
3 orange

Directions:

1. There are many types of kale available in the market. You can use any of them. In this recipe we have used curly kale.
2. Before you start juicing peeled out the oranges nicely.
3. Now switch on your blender and start juicing.
4. Serve with some ice cubes.

Kale-cium juice

Ingredients:

1 bunch of kale
4 stalks of celery
1 medium size apple
1 knuckle ginger

Directions:

1. A very simple Directions to make this juice.
2. Simply add all the ingredients in your blender.
3. Make sure that the kale is fresh enough as it is the main ingredient of this juice.
4. Serve and enjoy.

Sweet juice of kale

Ingredients:

4 and ½ cups chopped kale
3 cups grapes

Directions:

1. Use the Italian kale to make this juice. It will add an unique flavour in the juice.
2. If you want to make this juice cold then you can use frozen grapes for this recipe.
3. Add all the ingredients in your blender and turn it on.

Enjoy the sweet yet green juice.

The glowing juice

Ingredients:

2 cups of baby spinach
1 cup of arugula
1 medium size tomato
1 lemon
One small chunk of ginger
1 handful of basil
1 clove of garlic

Directions:

1. First blend the garlic and ginger in your blender and collect them in your mug.
2. Now place all the other items in the blender and start juicing.
3. Pour the juice with the blended garlic and ginger and stir properly.
4. Serve.

Baby spinach juice

Ingredients:

1 lemon
1-2 cups of baby spinach
¼ cabbage head
1 green apple
1 medium size beet

Directions:

1. Make sure you use fresh baby spinach and peeled out the lemon nicely.
2. Take your blender, put all the items and turn it on.
3. that is it.

Green with strawberries

Ingredients:

3-4 strawberries
1 small chunk of ginger
1 green apple
6 stalks of celery
2 carrots

Directions:

1. The Directions is very simple, just put all the items in your blender and switch it on.
2. This juice is not that much green but still it is very good for detoxing and weigh loss.

Spinach and cucumber juice

Ingredients:

2 cups of spinach
1 lemon
1 apple
Small chunk of ginger
1 lime
1 cucumber

Directions:

1. First make the lemon and lime juice.
2. You need to use unpeeled lemon for this juice.
3. Now simply add all the ingredients in your blender and start juicing.
4. Pour the juice in your mug.

Sweet kale juice with watermelon

Ingredients:

5 medium size carrots
1 bunch of parsley
Some leaves of Swiss chard
1/8 of a medium watermelon
15 medium leave of kale

Directions:

1. Peel carrots and cut the watermelon out of its skin and cut it into small cubes to fit in the blender.
2. Place all the ingredients in your blender and start juicing.
3. If your blender can't process the juice with the carrots you can make the carrot pulp separately.
4. Serve with some ice cubes. This is a great juice in the summer.

Juice master

Ingredients:

½ of a cucumber
2 sticks of celery
1 handful of spinach
1 tsp. of wheatgrass powder
1 slice of orange

Directions:

1. Simply adds all the items in your blender and start juicing.
2. Pour into a mug.
3. When drinking the juice take a bite of the orange slice.

Super-duper green juice

Ingredients:

2 small apples
Small piece of a carrot
½ stick- celery
1 large handful of varied green leaves like kale, parsley, spinach or whatever you get
½ in broccoli stem
½ slice of a raw beet root
Small slice of a lemon
½ ginger

Directions:

1. Cut all the ingredients into small pieces so your blender can take it.
2. Now place them into your blender and turn on it.
3. Pour the juice into a mug with some ice cubes.
4. You can store this for one day in an air tight jar.

Detox with Alfalfa Sprouts and watercress

Ingredients:

½ mug alfalfa sprouts
½ mug watercress
½ mug parsley
½ mug kale
2 apples
½ of a large pineapple
1 tsp. Wheat grass powder

Directions:

1. Juice all the ingredients in your blender and pour the juice in a mug.
2. Add the wheat grass powder in the last in your mug.
3. Stir nicely and enjoy.

Green evening juice

Ingredients:

½ stick- celery

1 chunk- cucumber
1 trickle of spinach
1 piece of peeled lime
2 fresh apples
½ ripe-avocado
½ small of a pineapple

Directions:

1. Place the avocado in your blender and all the other ingredients in the blender.
2. Now mix the blended avocado with the juice.
3. Serve and enjoy.

Supreme juice

Ingredients:

Spinach around 2 cup
Pear-1
Low fat yogurt- 2tbs.
½ of an avocado
Almond milk-1/2 cup
Chia seeds-1tbs.

Dlirections:

1. Make sure that you are using a ripe pear and low fat yogurt.
2. Place all the ingredients in your blender except the milk and yogurt and start juicing.
3. Pour the juice in a glass and then mix the yogurt and milk.
4. Stir properly and enjoy.

Kale juice with blueberries

Ingredients:

Blueberries-1 cup
1 apple
Cucumber-1
2 kale leaves
1 chunk of ginger

Directions:

1. Turn your blender on and put everything in it at once.
2. Juice it for two minutes.

Enjoy

Mean green

Ingredients:

Kale leave- 4 pieces
½ of a cucumber
1 orange
2 apples
¼ of a lemon (peeled)

Directions:

1. Wash the kale leafs properly before you put it in blender.
2. Put everything in blender.
3. Juice it for 3 minutes.

Enjoy

Green machine

Ingredients:

Spinach around 100 gram
Bitter ground-1 medium size
1 large size cucumber
Lemon juice-1 tsp.
A stalk celery
Green apple-1
Ginger – 1 large piece
½ of a lemon
A small pinch of pepper
Salt (optional)

Directions:

1. Wash everything properly.
2. Cut the apple into pieces.
3. Put everything in blender and juice it till it gets smooth.

Enjoy

Calm celery juice

Ingredients:

Celery -4 or 5 stalks
1 small size of beet
Spinach- 1 cup
Cilantro- 1 bunch
1 tsp. salt

Directions:

1. The spinach needs to be coarsely chopped and cut the beet in cubes.
2. Wash spinach and cilantro properly.
3. Put everything in blender and turn it on.
4. Juice it for 3 minutes.

Enjoy

Great cleanser juice

Ingredients:

Spinach-2 cups
Lemon juice
Lettuce leave- ½ cup
Cayenne pepper-1/4
1 pinch of salt
2 medium size green apples

Directions:

1. Wash lettuce leafs. Cut apples into pieces.
2. Put everything in blender and turn it on.
3. Juice it for 3 minutes.

Enjoy

Avocado and mango juice

Ingredients:

Avocado-1/2 (ripe)

1/3 cup of spinach
Mango-1/3 cup
Fresh lemon juice about ½ tsp.

Directions:

1. Put everything in blender and turn it on.
2. Juice for 3 minutes.
Enjoy

Creamy avocado juice

Ingredients:

½ ripe avocado
Fresh orange juice-1 cup
Low fat yogurt- 6 oz.

Directions:

1. Simply put everything in your blender and turn it on.
2. Juice it for 3-4 minutes.
Enjoy

Sweet avocado juice

Ingredients:

1 fresh ripe avocado
1 cup peer juice
Around 1 tbsp. honey
½ tsp of vanilla extract

Directions:

1. Put everything in blender at once.
2. Turn it on and juice for 4 minutes.
Enjoy.

Celery delight

Ingredients:

Celery-5 stalk
1 medium head of broccoli
½ of a cucumber
Small chunk of a ginger

Directions:

1. Put everything in your blender.
2. Turn it on and juice it for 3 minutes.

Enjoy

Celery and beet juice

Ingredients:

5 stalks of celery
2 cups chopped beet stalks
2 and ½ cups chopped romaine lettuce
1 fresh green apple

Directions:

1. Apple should be cut into pieces.
2. Put everything in blender.
3. Turn it on and juice it for 3 minutes.

Enjoy

Happiness of green

Ingredients:

5 stalks of celery
1 tsp. of honey
3 cups chopped red cabbage
3 medium size of carrots

Directions:

1. Carrots should be cut into pieces

2. Put everything in blender and turn it on.

3. Mix it for three minutes.

Enjoy.

Rainbow celery

Ingredients:

Rainbow chard- 2cups(copped)
Green apple-1 (peeled)
5/6 stalks of celery

Directions:

1. Put everything in your blender and turn it on.

2. Juice it for two minutes.

Enjoy

Celery with the taste of cilantro

Ingredients:

Cilantro- 1cup chopped
Cucumber-1
Celery-7
Kale- 2 and a half cup (chopped)
Apples -2

Directions:

1. Cut the apples into pieces.

2. Put everything in blender and turn it on.

3. Juice everything for two minutes.

Enjoy.

Full of green

Ingredients:

Bok Choy- 1 and ½ cups chopped
Beet- 1 small
1 handful of spinach
Celery- 5 stalks

Apple-1
2 leaf of parsley

Directions:

1. Cut the apples into pieces. Wash spinach before using.
2. Put everything in blender and turn it on. Juice it for two minutes.
Enjoy

Detox with celery

Ingredients:

Cantaloupe – 2 cups chopped
Lettuce-1/2 head
Celery- 7 stalks
Beets- 2 large
5 carrots
Red cabbage-2/3 of head

Directions:

1. Carrots need to be cut into pieces.
2. Put everything in blender and turn it on. Juice it for around 3 minutes.
Enjoy

Tropical twist

Ingredients:

Papaya -1 cup
Pineapple-1
Celery- 4 stalks

Directions:

1. You can also use mango for this juice if you don't love papaya.
2. Cut the fruits into cubes and place them with celery in the blender.
3. Collect the juice and serve with some ice cubes.

The chiller juice

Ingredients:

Cucumber- 1 large
Coconut- 8 and ½ ounce
Wheatgrass juice- around 3 ounces

Directions:

1. Use a young coconut for this juice.
2. First make the wheatgrass juice and add the coconut water with this.
3. Now make the cucumber juice and mix this with the first juice.
4. Serve and enjoy.

Refreshing juice

Ingredients:

Celery – 2 stalks
5 carrots
Thai coconut-1 (young coconut)
1 handful of broccoli

Directions:

1. Cut the carrots into pieces. Wash broccoli properly.
2. Put everything in blender and turn it on.
3. Juice for 3-4 minutes.
Enjoy

Alkaline juice

Ingredients:

Dandelion greens- 1 cup
Lemon- 1
Kale leaves- 2/3
Dandelion green -1 cup
Pea sprout-around ½ cup
Ginger- 1tbsp.
Cucumber-1
Celery-1

Parsley-1 cup
Apples-2

Directions:

1. Cut apples into pieces.
2. Put everything in blender and juice it for two minutes.

Enjoy

Romaine juice

Ingredients:

Romaine lettuce- 1 head
1 large handful of spinach
3 large green apples

Directions:

1. Wash lettuce properly
2. Cut apples into pieces.
3. Put everything in blender. Juice it for two-three minutes.

Enjoy

Cauliflower and romaine juice

Ingredients:

Cauliflower- ½ head
Carrots-3
Fennel-1 stalk
Romanian lettuce – 1 small head
Apple-1 small

Directions:

1. Cut apple and carrots into pieces.
2. Put everything in blender and juice for 4 minutes.

Enjoy

Wheat grass juice with lemonade

Ingredients:

Wheatgrass juice- 30 ml
Lemon juice -30 ml.

Directions:

1. You can make the lemon juice with your hands by only squeezing the lemons.
2. Now feed the wheatgrass into your blender. Fill the blender with the wheatgrass a little amount once a time. It will be then easy to get the juice.
3. Mix the lemon juice and wheatgrass juice properly.
4. Serve and enjoy.

Minty wheatgrass juice

Ingredients:

Mint leaves- 1 handful
¼ of a Medium size pineapple
Wheatgrass juice- 30 ml

Directions:

1. Cut pineapple into pieces.
2. Put everything in blender and juice it for 3 minutes.
Enjoy

Special cleanser juice

Ingredients:

Wheatgrass juice- 30 ml
1 handful of parsley
Carrots-3
½ of a beetroot
Celery- 2 stalks
½ of a lemon (peeled)
Some mint leaves for serving

Directions:

1. Put everything in blender.

2. Juice it for three minutes.
Enjoy.

Energy drink

Ingredients:

30 ml of wheatgrass juice
1 lemon
1 carrot
1 pink grapefruit
1 fresh orange

Directions:

1. Carrot and Orange need to be cut into pieces.
2. Put everything in blender and juice it.
Enjoy

Mint breath

Ingredients:

1 large handful of meant leaves
Wheatgrass juice- 30 ml
Peppermint extract-1/2 tsp.(organic)

Directions:

1. Wash mint and grass properly.
2. Put everything in blender and juice it till it gets smooth.
Enjoy

Ginger shot

Ingredients:

1 slice of lemon
Water-300 ml
Wheatgrass juice-30ml
Fresh ginger-1-2 cm

Directions:

1. Put everything in blender and juice for 3 minutes. Enjoy.

Green day

Ingredients:

Pineapple-1/2
Cucbers-2
Some leaves of mint

Directions:

1. Take your blender and simply place all the ingredients there.
2. After juicing pour the juice into a mug.

Orange and parsley juice

Ingredients:

Oranges-4/5
1 bunch of parsley

Directions:

1. You must need to peel oranges otherwise the juice will taste bitter.
2. Now place the peeled oranges and parsley into your blender and start juicing. It will be better if you make the juices separately. Like first make the orange juice then parsley juice.
3. Make sure that you have cleaned your blender.

Oh green!

Ingredients:

Cucbers-3
Kale-2 stalk
1 handful of parsley
Spinach-1/2 bunch
Swiss chard-1/2 bunch
½ lime(you can also use lemons)
Stevia(according to your taste)

Directions:

1. the Directions for this juice is really very simple. All you need is to place the items in your blender and start juicing.
2. Cut the ingredients in small pieces so it can fit in the chutes of the blender.
3. Serve immediately.

Swiss chard juice

Ingredients:

Swiss chard-6/8 leaves
Kale-6 leaves
Honeydew- ½
Cantaloupe-1/2
2 fresh green apples

Directions:

1. Put everything in blender and juice for 3 minutes.
Enjoy.

Swiss chard with ginger

Ingredients:

Swiss chard-6 leaves
¼ of a lemon
Carrots-2
Cabagge-1
Apples-2

Directions:

1. Put everything in blender and juice for 3 minutes.
Enjoy.

Green combo

Ingredients:

Green apples-2
2 cups of spinach
Swiss chard-6 to 8 leaves
Cucumber-1
Fennel bulb-1/2
Basil around 1 bunch

Directions:

1. Cut apples into pieces.
2. Put everything in blender and juice for 3 minutes.
Enjoy.

Green jug

Ingredients:

1 fresh green apple
1 lime
Cilantro-4 leaves(chopped)
Cucumbers-2
Pepper-1
Small handful of spinach

Directions:

1. You need to remove the ribs and seeds from the pepper.
2. Turn on your blender and add all the items there.
3. Serve with some ice cubes.

Spinach and fennel juice

Ingredients:

3 cups full spinach
Celery stalks-3
1 large cucumber
Fennel bulb-1

Directions:

1. Put everything in blender and juice for 3 minutes. Enjoy.

Green fruity mix

Ingredients:

Coconut water-1cup
Strawberries-10
½ of a pear
1 green apple
2 cups kale
2 cups spinach
2 cups of beet greens

Directions:

1. Cut the green tops of the strawberries and use unsweetened coconut water.
2. Measure the items in a measuring cup and then put them in your blender.
3. Collect the juice in a mug and enjoy.

Green power juice

Ingredients:

Parsley-2 cups
¼ of a small red onion
Celery-2 stalks
Cucumber-1
2 green tomatoes(raw tomatoes)

Directions:

1. Put everything in blender and juice for 3 minutes. Enjoy.

Green power juice

Ingredients:

Swiss chard-3 cups
1 cup of green cabbage

Carrots-2
Beets-2
2 fresh green apple
Pears-1

Directions:

1. Put everything in blender and juice for 3 minutes.
Enjoy.

Green chard with pineapple

Ingredients:

Swiss chard leaves-3 cups
Banana- 2cups
Pineapple chunks-2 cups
Mango chunks-1 cup
1 cup of water

Directions:

1. Bananas need to be smashed.

2. Put everything in blender with water.

3. Turn it on and juice it for 4 minutes.
Enjoy.

Green chard with pineapple

Ingredients:

Swiss chard leaves-3 cups
Bananan-2cups(smashed)
Pineapple chunks-2 cups
Mango chunks-1 cup
1 cup of water

Quick and simple green juice

Ingredients:

12 ounces of filtered water
Wheatgrass powder-1 tbsp.
Spirulina powder

Directions:

1. You don't need a blender for this.
2. Just take a mug and there mix the powders with water.

Pineapple and kale combo

Ingredients:

Kale leafs-3
1 tsp. of honey
½ of lemon
1 green apple
1 cup frozen pineapple

Direction:

1. Chopped the vegetables and peel the lemon.
2. Now take your blender and start juicing.
3. Serve and enjoy.

Sweet cucumber juice

Ingredients:

Spinach-4 handful
Apples-4
Cucumbers-2

Directions:

1. Simply place all the ingredients in your blender and turn it on.
2. Collect the juice in a mug and serve with some ice cubes.

Mint breath

Ingredients:

Small handful of spinach
½ of a ripe pineapple
Cucumber-2
Mint-1 bunch

Directions:

1. Take your blender and run all the items there.
2. In a mug serve this juice with some mint leaves.

Green island

Ingredients:

Lemon-1
Lettuce – 2 heads
1 handful of kale
Green apples-4
Small handful of parsley

Directions:

1. Chopped the ingredients and first extract the juice from the lemon.
2. Now add all these in the blender and make the juice.
3. Serve and enjoy.

Sunshine juice

Ingredients:

Pink grape fruit-1
Oranges-2
Mint-1 bunch
Lettuce-1 head

Directions:

1. Peel the oranges and grapefruit.
2. Now run the entire items in your blender.
3. Serve with some mint leaves.

Green shot

Ingredients:

Cucumbers-2
Apples-2
Limes-2
6/7 leaves of kale

Parsley-several sprigs
4/5 leaves of mint

Directions:

1. You will need to follow a simple Directions to make this juice. First remove the skin from the limes
2. You will run all these ingredients in your blender.
3. Collect the juice in a mug and enjoy.

Cucumber and pear juice

Ingredients:

Pears-3
Cucumber-1
½ bunch of fresh parsley
Some mint leaves
1tsp. honey

Directions:

1. Cut the fruits into small cubes so that it can fit in your blender.
2. Place the ingredients in your blender and switch it on.
3. Serve and enjoy.

Spicy green

Ingredients:

1. 2 cups chopped frozen pineapple
2. Kale leaves-5/6
3. 1 large cucumber
4. 1 jalapeno

Directions:

1. If you find it too much spicy then use ½ of the jalapeno.
2. Run all these ingredients in your blender and enjoy.

Green grape juice

Ingredients:

Green grapes-2 cups
½ of a large cucumber
1 fresh green apple
½ piece of a ginger
Chard leaves-6

Direction:

1. Simply add all the ingredients in your blender and switch it on.
2. Serve and enjoy.

Green deep

Ingredients:

Green apple-1
Collard leaves-6
Celery ribs-2
½ of a lemon(peeled)
1/8 of a fennel blub
1 cucumber

Directions:

1. Simply put all the ingredients in your blender.
2. Serve with some ice cubes.

Clean green juice

Ingredient:

Zucchini-1
Pears-3
Fennel blub-1/8
Broccoli florets-4
1 handful of spinach

Directions:

1. First clean all the ingredients properly.

2. Run all the ingredients in your blender.

Kale and grapefruit

Ingredients:

Kale leaves-4
Apples-2
½ of a grapefruit
1 orange(peeled)

Directions:

1. Cut the fruits.
2. Place the fruits with the kale leaves and start juicing.
Enjoy.

Chard and orange juice

Ingredients:

Swiss chard-3
10 parsley leaves9(chopped)
1 fresh green apple
Oranges-2
½ of a large cucumber

Directions:

1. Chop up the parsley leaves and Swiss chard.
2. Now turn on your blender place the ingredients.
3. Collect the juice in a mug.

Watermelon juice

Ingredients:

2 cup watermelon
Aplles-2 piece
½ of a lemon(peeled)
Kale -4 leafs

Directions:

1. Put everything in your blender.
2. Serve immediately.

Celery and Arugula juice

Ingredients:

Arugula-1 handful
2 Celery stalks
½ of a lime
2 cup watermelon(cubed)

Directions:

1. Simply put everything in your blender.
2. Serve and enjoy.

Cream of green

Ingredients:

Avocado-1
Bannan-1 (frozen)
1 small piece of orange
1 cup of fresh spinach
1 cup vanilla milk

Directions:

1. Remove the pits from the avocado.
2. Use unsweetened vanilla milk.
3. Run all the ingredients in your blender.

Spinach-berry juice

Ingredients:

Spinach-2 cup
1 piece of banana
3 cups of frozen berries
¼ cup of raw nuts

Directions:

1. Peel the banana.
2. Except the raw nut place all the ingredients in your blender and turn it on.
3. Place the nuts over the juice and serve.

Pomegranate and spinach juice

Ingredients:

1 cup pomegranate seeds
1 cup fresh orange juice
2 cup chopped orange juice

Directions:

1. First make the orange juice in the blender and then collect it in a mug.
2. Now put other ingredients in the blender.
3. Collect the juice and mix with the orange juice.

Peachy green juice

Ingredients:

2 cups of Bok Choy
2 cup peach
2 cups almond milk

Directions:

1. You have to use unsweetened almond milk.
2. First make juice of the pear and Bok Choy.
3. Then mix the almond milk with the juice and enjoy.

Pineapple-spinach-avocado combo

Ingredients:

1 piece of avocado
2cup spinach
2 cup frozen pineapple
2 cup unsweetened coconut water

Directions:

1. It is very easy to make this juice. Just put all the ingredients in your blender and start juicing.
2. Serve and enjoy.

Lemonade of Dande

Ingredients:

Dandelion Greens-1cup
Lime juice-1 cup
Kale-1 cup
Honey-2 tsp

Directions:

1. Wash your blender first
2. Add all the ingredients in the blender and turn it on.
3. That is it .Enjoy

Green Crush of Beet

Ingredients:

Beet greens-1 cup
Romaine lettuce-1 cup
Water-2 cup
Banana-3 pieces
Sugar-2 tsp

Directions:

1. 1. All of the green ingredients should be fresh.
2. Add all the ingredients in the blender and turn it on.
3. That is it.
Enjoy.

Swiss Chard Refresher

Ingredients:

Green apple-2 piece (sliced)
Swiss Chard-1 cup
Mint-2 or 3 leaves
Water-1 cup
Ginger flavor -2 tsp

Directions:

1. Add all the ingredients in the blender .
2. Make sure all the ingredients are fresh.
3. Thats it. Now enjoy.

Pummelo Twist of Orange

Ingredients:

Orange juice-1 cup
Pummelo-1 cup
Ginger -1 tsp
Baby spinach-1/2 cup
Mint-1 handful

Directions:

1. Turn Your blender on and blend orange juice with baby spinach
2. Now add the other items and blend it again for two minutes .
3. Remember all the green ingredients have to be fresh.
4. Now enjoy it.

Sprinkles of Cabbage

Ingredients:

Green grapes juice-1 cup
Cabbage-1 cup
Mustard greens- 2 or 3 leaves
Kale- 1 cup

Directions:

1. Turn your blender on and blend green grapes juice.
2. Now add all the other ingredients and blend it for three minutes.
3. That is all. Now enjoy

Fountain of Green

Ingredients:

Oat milk -1 cup
Baby spinach-1 cup
Romaine lettuce-1/2 cup
Cilantro-1 or 2 leaves
Carrot tops-1 stalk
Honey-2 tsp

Directions:

1. Keep the blender clean before using it.
2. Add all the ingredients in the blender and blend it for three minutes.
3. Now enjoy.

Broccoli with banana

Ingredients

Broccoli-1 cup
Banana-2 pieces
Water-3/4th cup
Chard-1/2 cup
Almond milk-3/4th cup

Directions:

1. First of all mix all the liquids together.
2. Now add all the ingredients in the blender and blend it for two   minutes
3. You can use ice if you want it cold. It is up to you enjoy.

Lemonade crush with Spinach

Ingredients:

Lime juice-1 cup
Spinach-1 cup
Collard-1 cup
Water-1 cup
Honey or Sugar-2 tsp

Directions:

1. Make the blender clean before using it.
2. Now add all the ingredients together.
3. You can add two-three cubes of ice.
Enjoy

Turnip greens with pomegranate

Ingredients:

Turnip greens- 2 cups
Pomegranate juice- 1 cup
Ginger-1 tsp
Chard-1/2 cup
Water-1 cup

Directions:

1.Add all the ingredients together in the blender and turn it on.
2.Use two cubes of ice.
3.Thats it .Enjoy

Kale- Pomegranate punch

Ingredients:

Pomegranate juice- 1 cup
Kale-1 cup
Ginger-1 tsp
Mint-1 handful
Water-3/4th cup

Directions:

1. Keep your blender clean.
2. Now add all the ingredients in the blender and blend it.
3. That is it. Now enjoy.

Carrot lovers smoothie

Ingredients:

Baby carrot-1 cup
Carrot tops-3 stalk
Cabbage-1 cup
Turnip green-1 cup
Water-1 cup
Honey-2 tsp

Directions:

1. Take the carrots and mix it with spinach.
2. Remember all the green ingredients needs to be fresh.
3. Now put everything and blend for two minutes.

Spinach covered with chocolate smoothie

Ingredients:

Spinach-1 cup
Cinnamon-1 tsp
Cocoa powder-3 tsp
Almond milk-1 cup (unsweetened)
Cherry-1 cup

Directions:

1. First mix the powders with milk.
2. Now add all the ingredients in the blender and blend it.
3. Add three cubes of ice. It is up to you.
Enjoy

Avocado-Kale smoothie

Ingredients:

Avocado-1/2 amount
Almond milk-1 cup
Kale-1 cup
Cherry-1 cup

Directions:

1. Take the kale and mix it with almond milk.
2. Now add all the ingredients together in the blend.
3. That is it.
Enjoy

Cabbage Lanterns

Ingredients:

Cabbage-2 cup
Oat milk-1 cup
Baby carrots-1/2 cup
Cilantro- 1 handful
Honey-2 tsp

Directions:

1. Turn on the blender and add all the all the ingredients together
2. Make sure the carrots are fresh.
3. That is .Enjoy

Smoothie of Broccoli and Cherry

Ingredients:

Broccoli-1 cup
Cherry-1 cup
Lime juice-1/2 cup
Honey-1 tsp
Cinnamon-1 tsp

Directions:

1. Mix lime juice and cherry together in the blender.
2. Add all the ingredients together and blend it for two minutes.
3. That is it.

Enjoy

Choco Collards

Ingredients:

Collards-1 cup
Cocoa powder-3 tsp
Cinnamon-1 tsp
Banana-1 piece

Directions:

1. Clean the blender before use.
2. Now add all the ingredients together and blend it for two minutes.
3. That is it .Enjoy.

Peach Green Smoothie

Ingredients:

Peach-1 piece, pealed
Cinnamon-1 tsp
Spinach-1 cup
Arugula-1 cup
Water-1 cup

Directions:

1. Firstly, take spinach and blend it them together.
2. Now add all the other ingredients into the blender and blend it again.
3. Use two cubes of ice to make the smoothie cold.
4. This is it.

Enjoy.

Choy Choco

Ingredients:

Coconut water-1 cup
Cinnamon-1tsp
Cherry-1/2 cup
Bok choy-1 cup, sliced
Spinach-1 cup

Directions:

1. Firstly, take the spinach and coconut water and blend them together.
2. Now add the other things in the blender and blend it again.
3. Remember that you need to take out cherry pits before you make the smoothie.
Enjoy

Parsley with Mixed cherry Smoothie

Ingredients:

Parsley-1 cup
Mixed berry-1 cup
Water-1 cup
Honey-2 tsp
Broccoli-1 cup

Directions:

1. Always keep the blender clean.
2. Now add all the ingredients into the blender and blend it.
3. That is it. Enjoy.

Celery with orange smoothie

Ingredients:

Orange juice-1 cup
Aloe vera-1/2 cup
Celery-1 cup,sliced
Water-1 cup
Mint-1 handful
Ginger-1 tsp

Directions:

1. Keep your blender clean and mix orange juice with aloe vera.
2. Now add all the ingredients together and blend it for two minutes.
3. That is all. Enjoy.

Swiss chard jazz

Ingredients:

Swiss chard-1 cup
Blue berry-1 cup
Mixed berry-1 cup
Kiwi-1 piece
Spinach-2 cups
Lime juice-1 cup

Directions:

1. Mix the lime juice with kiwi and spinach first.
2. Now add all the ingredients together in the blender and blend it for two minutes.
3. That is all . Enjoy.

Dandelion with mango

Ingredients:

Dandelion-2 cups
Mango-2 cups
Spinach-1 cup
Milk-1 cup
Cinnamon-1 tsp

Directions:

1. Keep your blender clean and mix milk with mango.
2. Now add all the ingredients together and blend it for two minutes.
3. That is all. Enjoy.

Sprouts sizzles

Ingredients:

Sprouts-2 cup
Lime juice-1 cup
Spinach-1/2 cup
Mints-1 handful
Honey-2 tsp

Directions:

1. Firstly, add mints and sprouts together and blend it .
2. Now add all the ingredients and blend it for three minutes.
3. That is all. Enjoy.

Honey Green Veg

Ingredients:

Spinach-2 cups
Broccoli-1 cup
Cabbage-1/2 cup
Sweet potatoes-1 piece
Honey-3 tsp
Almond milk-1 cup

Directions:

1. Mixed the milk with the sweet potato and honey and blend it.
2. Now add all the ingredients together and blend it until it becomes thick
3. Boil the sweet potatoes, before blending. Enjoy.

Romaine lettuce with peach and Avocado

Ingredients:

Romaine lettuce-1 cup
Peach-1 cup
Avocado- 1 amount
Honey-2 tsp
Ginger-1 tsp
Mints-2 tsp

Directions:

1. Firstly add all the ingredients together into the blender and blend.
2. You can use frozen fruits to make it cold.
3. That is all .Enjoy.

Bonus

Beet greens with mango crush

Ingredients:

Beet greens-1 cup
Mango-1 amount, pealed
Honey-2 tsp
Mint-2 or 3 leaves

Directions:

1. Firstly, add the whole ingredients together and blend it.
2. Add two ice cubes for making it cold.
3. That is all. Enjoy .

Strawberry with Arugula smoothie

Ingredients:

Strawberry-1 cup
Arugula-1 cup
Cucumber-1 cup
Spinach-1/2 cup
Mints-1 handful
Water-3/4th cup

Description:

1. Mixed the strawberry, mints and the water together in the blender.
2. Now,add all the ingredients together and blend it again for two minutes.
3. You can use frozen strawberry to make the smoothie cold. Enjoy

Conclusion

The book 365 days of Green Smoothies Recipes is mainly designed to make each and every cook book lovers have an enjoyment to make awesome smoothies at home. The cook book includes the best recipes which the writer had tested. The book is well printed with top class smoothies. Some sample recipes are:

Spring with Green Smoothie

Pear apple fun

Arugula smoothie

These are few from the best recipes which the book contains. The book has the best and most efficient of all kind of steps that a housewife needs to present her magic in the kitchen. Everyone can enjoy the best green smoothies and that is the moto of the book. Hope you all will like this.

Thank you again for purchasing this book!

Finally, if you enjoyed this book, please take the time to share your thoughts and post a review on Amazon. It'd be greatly appreciated!

Feel free to contact me at emma.katie@outlook.com

Check out more books by Emma Katie at:

www.amazon.com/author/emmakatie

www.ingramcontent.com/pod-product-compliance
Lightning Source LLC
Chambersburg PA
CBHW081826280526
45789CB00007B/2365